Fall Prevention and Geriatric Nursing

Fall Prevention and Geriatric Nursing

Guest Editors

Cristina Lavareda Baixinho
Andreia Costa
Adriana Henriques

MDPI

Basel • Beijing • Wuhan • Barcelona • Belgrade • Novi Sad • Cluj • Manchester

Guest Editors
Cristina Lavareda Baixinho
Nursing Research Innovation and Development Centre of Lisbon (CIDNUR)
University of Lisbon
Lisbon
Portugal

Andreia Costa
Nursing Research Innovation and Development Centre of Lisbon (CIDNUR)
University of Lisbon
Lisbon
Portugal

Adriana Henriques
Nursing Research Innovation and Development Centre of Lisbon (CIDNUR)
University of Lisbon
Lisbon
Portugal

Editorial Office
MDPI AG
Grosspeteranlage 5
4052 Basel, Switzerland

This is a reprint of the Special Issue, published open access by the journal *Healthcare* (ISSN 2227-9032), freely accessible at: https://www.mdpi.com/journal/healthcare/special_issues/16UV7F2423.

For citation purposes, cite each article independently as indicated on the article page online and as indicated below:

Lastname, A.A.; Lastname, B.B. Article Title. *Journal Name* **Year**, *Volume Number*, Page Range.

ISBN 978-3-7258-7923-6 (Hbk)
ISBN 978-3-7258-7924-3 (PDF)
https://doi.org/10.3390/books978-3-7258-7924-3

Contents

healthcare

MDPI

torial

all Prevention and Geriatric Nursing

istina Lavareda Baixinho [1,2,*], Maria Adriana Henriques [1,3,4] and Andreia Costa [1,3,4]

1 Nursing Research Innovation and Development Centre of Lisbon (CIDNUR), School of Nursing, Universidade de Lisboa, 1600-096 Lisbon, Portugal
2 Center for Innovative Care and Health Technology (ciTechcare), 2414-016 Leiria, Portugal
3 Instituto de Saúde Ambiental, Faculdade de Medicina, Universidade de Lisboa, 1649-028 Lisbon, Portugal
4 Laboratório Associado TERRA, Universidade de Lisboa, 1349-017 Lisbon, Portugal
* Correspondence: crbaixinho@esel.pt

1. Introduction

Falls among older people remain one of the most pressing and persistent public health challenges worldwide [1]. Given the increased life expectancy, and prevalence of disability, dependency, and comorbidities in this ageing population, there is a high risk that this will become a pandemic.

On the other hand, as populations age the consequences of falls increase, ranging from physical injury and loss of functional independence to psychological distress, fear of falling, social isolation, and increased mortality, posing significant challenges not only to individuals and families but also to healthcare systems and societies [2,3]. Falls are a leading cause of injury-related hospitalizations among older persons and contribute substantially to escalating healthcare costs, long-term care admissions, and diminished quality of life [2].

The growing proportion of older adults, many living with multimorbidity, frailty, cognitive impairment, and social vulnerability, demands a critical rethinking of health, social, and urban policies to support healthy ageing [2–4]. While fall prevention is often framed as an individual responsibility, this perspective risks overlooking structural, educational, and systemic barriers that limit older adults' capacity to engage in effective prevention strategies, such as low health literacy, unequal access to preventive services, and environments that are not age-friendly [4].

Despite robust evidence supporting effective fall prevention strategies [5], many health systems continue to prioritise secondary and tertiary care over proactive, primary prevention [4,5]. This imbalance contributes to missed opportunities for early risk identification, timely interventions, and sustained behaviour change. Moreover, fall risk is inherently multidimensional, encompassing physical, psychological, environmental, social, and behavioural factors [3,5]. Interventions are therefore necessarily complex, often requiring interdisciplinary collaboration, individualised assessment, and long-term follow-up, which can be difficult to consistently implement in real-world settings [4,5].

Within this complex geriatric syndrome, geriatric nursing plays a central role. Nurses are uniquely positioned across care settings—community, primary care, hospitals, long-term care facilities, and home care—to identify fall risks, implement evidence-based interventions, educate older adults and caregivers, work with municipal councils local for the creation of safer environments, and advocate for national health policies that prioritise this public health problem. Their close, continuous contact with older persons enables a holistic understanding of patients' functional abilities, fears, preferences, and lived experiences, all of which are essential for effective fall prevention.

This Special Issue on Fall Prevention and Geriatric Nursing aims to contribute to this critical field by bringing together high-quality research and reviews that advance knowledge and practice. The published articles explore innovative, person-centred, and context-sensitive interventions for fall prevention and risk management in different life contexts, and models of education and training for health professionals and caregivers.

We invite nurses, researchers, educators, and healthcare professionals to explore the published articles. Together, we can strengthen the role of geriatric nursing and contribute meaningfully to healthier ageing and safer societies.

2. Recent Developments in the Field

A review of the literature reveals that research in the area of falls has been productive, with several meta-analyses and other robust studies that have uncovered knowledge about fall risk factors [6–10], development of predictive models [11–13], and preventive measures [14–17], aimed at controlling the risk, prevalence, and severity of injuries.

Although the growing body of research has deepened understanding of falls, it has also made it harder to identify, appraise, and synthesise evidence on risk factors—both in terms of methodological quality and in translating findings into consistent assessment and intervention pathways. Falls arise from multiple interacting factors, making them a complex public health problem that requires multidimensional, person-centred interventions tailored to each individual's risk profile.

A major step forward has been the consolidation of international guidance in the World Guidelines for Falls Prevention and Management for Older Adults, developed by an international expert panel under the auspices of the Global Falls Guidelines Group. These guidelines recommend a structured pathway: (1) case-finding and initial screening to identify older adults at increased risk (e.g., previous falls, gait or balance impairment, fear of falling); (2) a comprehensive multifactorial assessment for those at higher risk; and (3) the delivery of targeted, evidence-based interventions with ongoing review and follow-up [5].

One of the greatest challenges in both clinical practice and research has been the availability and use of fall risk assessment instruments. Identifying a tool that is valid and reliable, with strong predictive accuracy and an acceptable balance between false positives and false negatives, has proven difficult; as a result, clinical services often rely on a wide variety of instruments, limiting comparability and consistency in decision-making.

The proposed World Guidelines to organise assessment and decision-making centre around three key questions (3KQ) [5]: can we solve this problem with the use of an instrument that has a higher sensitivity, it is easy to use, and does it require minimal time for healthcare professionals to adopt this new opportunistic screening method?

The World Guidelines propose organising assessment and clinical decision-making around three key questions (3KQ): 1—Have you fallen in the past year? 2—Do you feel unsteady when standing or walking? 3—Do you have worries about falling? [5]. This approach can help address current difficulties in fall risk evaluation by using a brief screening tool with high sensitivity that is easy to apply and takes little time for healthcare professionals. By reducing complexity and time burden, the 3KQ can also increase professionals' adherence to opportunistic screening, improving early identification of older adults who need more detailed assessment and targeted interventions.

The multifactorial assessment of people with a high risk of falls is essential to determine the individual combination of modifiable risk factors (such as strength and balance deficits, medication effects, orthostatic hypotension/syncope, vision problems, environmental hazards, footwear, cognition, and continence) [5–11] and is addressed by delivering tailored interventions matched to the identified risks (education on fall preven-

https://doi.org/10.3390/healthcare14050630

tion, progressive balance and strength exercise, medication review/deprescribing where appropriate, management of cardiovascular causes, environmental modifications, and education) [5,14–17], alongside clear follow-up to review adherence, outcomes, and any new risks [5].

Education for fall prevention, together with exercise, remains central to effective risk reduction [5]. In hospital settings, the single and multifactorial approaches for prevention included staff and patient education, environmental modifications, assistive devices, policies and systems, rehabilitation, medication management, and management of cognitive impairment [14].

To prevent falls among community-dwelling older adults, evidence from a minimum of 1–2 years is beneficial, and interventions include supervised, long-duration balance/resistance and group Tai Chi, whole-body vibration, high-intensity/dose education or cognitive behavioural therapy, and comprehensive multifactorial assessment with targeted treatment plus home hazard assessment and the provision of education [18].

The strongest evidence supports exercise programmes that challenge balance and build strength, delivered with adequate dose and progression (commonly around $\geq$3 h per week over several months), as these are most likely to improve postural control and functional capacity and reduce falls [5,18–22]. Recent practice has increasingly focused on tailoring exercise to individual needs and conditions (e.g., frailty, Parkinson's disease, stroke), combining supervised and home-based formats [18,20], and incorporating behaviour-change strategies (such as goal setting, feedback, and problem-solving) to strengthen motivation and adherence [5,21–23].

In parallel, technology has advanced: wearable sensors and smartphone-based assessments can support gait and balance monitoring, quantify activity, and track response to interventions, although successful implementation still depends on usability, equitable access, data governance, and clear integration into clinical pathways [23–25].

3. Knowledge Gaps

As previously noted, research on falls has been highly productive in recent years. However, the magnitude of the problem—and its potential to escalate rapidly to near-pandemic levels—underscores the ongoing need for rigorous, robust studies in this field.

Regarding risk factor assessment, much of the current research remains strongly oriented towards the biomedical model, prioritising the identification of biophysiological determinants of falls [3,5,7,26,27]. Given the often multifactorial nature of falls, future fall risk assessment studies should also incorporate psychosocial, environmental, and individual behavioural factors, enabling an understanding of their association with each other.

Studies recommend education for fall prevention as a cost-effective intervention, but they also highlight persistent challenges with adherence. More recently, research has begun to explore psychoeducational and behaviour change interventions aimed at improving adherence to safety behaviours. However, findings remain inconclusive, possibly reflecting a shortage of in-depth studies examining how older adults, health and social care professionals, and informal caregivers make decisions about maintaining safety and preventing accidents. For example, a systematic review assessing the benefits and harms of psychological and educational interventions to prevent falls among community-dwelling older adults concluded that the evidence for individual psychological interventions or education delivered as a stand-alone strategy is of low or very low certainty [26].

Similarly, there is persistent uncertainty about which behaviour-change techniques most effectively promote long-term participation in exercise and uptake of home-safety actions, and how these strategies should be tailored to individual differences in cognition, culture, fear of falling, social support, and other psychosocial factors [5,26]. Evidence is

https://doi.org/10.3390/healthcare14050630

also comparatively limited for people living with cognitive impairment or dementia, where the safest and most effective intervention "packages" remain unclear and must balance autonomy and mobility with supervision needs, carer burden, and outcomes beyond falls alone (e.g., agitation, function, quality of life) [27].

In institutional settings, multifactorial fall prevention programmes implemented in hospitals and long-term care facilities have produced mixed and sometimes modest effects. This variability suggests that multifactorial interventions should not be treated as a single, uniform approach. Instead, there is a need to disentangle which specific components (and which combinations) are responsible for observed benefits, whether effects differ by resident/patient profiles (e.g., frailty, cognitive impairment, post-acute illness, history of falls, medication burden), and how implementation is shaped by organisational and environmental conditions [5,14,16,26].

Even in areas where there is solid evidence of the impact of the intervention, such as balance and strength exercise, it seems that important knowledge gaps remain in translating efficacy into sustainable impact at scale. In practice, programme effectiveness is likely to depend not only on the content of the intervention (e.g., medication review, strength and balance training, mobility assistance, continence care, vision/footwear assessment, environmental hazard reduction), but also on the context in which it is delivered. Organisational factors such as staffing ratios and skill mix, staff training and turnover, teamwork and communication, leadership support, and the extent to which mobility is encouraged versus restricted can all influence whether interventions are applied consistently and safely [26,28,29].

Similarly, environmental and design features—such as bed height, lighting, flooring, clutter and layout, availability of handrails, accessibility of call bells and toilets, and use of assistive technologies—may enable or undermine safer mobility. Clarifying "what works, for whom, and under what conditions" is therefore essential to improve programme targeting, standardise implementation with fidelity, and guide institutions in allocating resources to the components most likely to deliver meaningful reductions in falls and fall-related harm [14,16,26].

Further uncertainty persists regarding the optimal "dose" and progression of exercise and the degree of personalisation required for those with multimorbidity, pain, severe frailty, or neurological conditions, without diluting effectiveness [14–17,27].

Additional gaps include the need for clearer evidence on which home modifications deliver meaningful risk reduction across different housing contexts and individual risk profiles, including for tenants and low-income households, and on how personalised home-environment interventions, smart home technologies, and long-term adaptability influence both the prevalence of falls and the nature and severity of related injuries [30,31].

An often overlooked yet critical dimension of falls is the fear of falling. Even in the absence of previous falls, fear can lead to activity restriction, physical deconditioning, reduced social participation, and a subsequent increase in actual fall risk. Addressing fear of falling requires not only physical interventions but also psychological support, empowerment, and confidence-building strategies—areas in which nursing-led interventions have demonstrated considerable promise [3,5,6,28,29].

A key knowledge gap concerns the optimal content, delivery, and impact of education and training to advance fall prevention, including how best to educate older adults and informal caregivers while strengthening health professionals' competencies through continuous development in fall risk assessment, multifactorial interventions, communication strategies, and interprofessional collaboration [5,28]. Further evidence is needed on how to prepare nurses and other professionals to translate evidence into practice and adapt interventions effectively across diverse cultural, social, and care contexts.

https://doi.org/10.3390/healthcare14050630

4. Contributions of the Special Issue

By fostering interdisciplinary dialogue and disseminating evidence-based practices, this Special Issue seeks to support the development of more effective and sustainable approaches to fall prevention. Ultimately, reducing falls and their consequences is not only about preventing injuries—it is about preserving autonomy, dignity, and quality of life for older adults.

Together, the studies of these Editions expand current knowledge on falls by strengthening risk identification, clarifying modifiable clinical and psychosocial correlates, and adding context-specific evidence across care settings and health-system levels.

In stroke rehabilitation, Hong et al. (contribution 1) contribute by testing the predictive validity of the Johns Hopkins Fall Risk Assessment Tool (JHFRAT) in an older, clinically complex population, reinforcing the importance of structured risk stratification to inform prevention planning during recovery phases in which mobility, cognition, and supervision needs can fluctuate. These results can aid nurses working in rehabilitation wards in more effectively utilising JHFRAT outcomes for post-stroke older patients with a low handgrip strength and contribute to the development of more appropriate fall prevention strategies for high-risk patients.

The single-centre, observational, retrospective study of patients aged 70 years and over admitted to the emergency department (ED) of the University Hospital of Guadeloupe, developed by Simo-Tabue et al. (contribution 2) contribute to the evidence that polypharmacy is meaningfully linked to hospitalisation among older adults presenting with falls, highlighting medication burden as a key, actionable factor to address through medication review, and deprescribing-oriented approaches after fall-related emergency visits. The authors strongly suggest that a regular review of drug prescriptions is essential to reduce polypharmacy in older adults.

In the community, Pereira et al. (contribution 3) deepen understanding of the interrelationship between falls, fear of falling, and depressive symptoms, supporting a more integrated view in which psychological health and fall risk are intertwined and suggesting that effective prevention may need to combine physical risk reduction with attention to emotional and behavioural consequences such as activity restriction and loss of confidence. The researchers observed depressive symptoms in 18.3% of the participants, with 90.5% of the participants reporting a fear of falling (FOF). More than half (63.0%) experienced falls, with 49.5% occurring in the last year. Factors such as the female gender, negative health perceptions, and functional dependence were associated with depressive symptoms. Adjusted analyses indicated that both a fear of falling (FOF) ($B = 0.043$; $p = 0.012$) and a history of falls ($B = 0.725$; $p = 0.015$) were associated with depressive symptoms. Based on the results, the authors call for targeted interventions to improve mental and physical health.

Miura and Kanoya (contribution 4) conducted a narrative review of studies published between 2019 and 2024 on fall risk assessment and prevention in nursing homes. Their findings synthesise and interpret the current evidence base, mapping commonly used assessment tools and preventive strategies and highlighting the multifactorial nature of falls in institutional settings, where resident frailty, cognitive impairment, environmental hazards, and care routines interact. The authors note that fall risk assessment in nursing homes still lacks practical indicators tailored to the specific characteristics and workflows of long-term care facilities, reinforcing the need for coordinated, team-based, multifactorial prevention rather than isolated measures. They also emphasise that, although a range of digital technologies has been proposed for fall prevention, there is a shortage of empirical studies demonstrating their effectiveness and feasibility in real-world nursing home practice.

https://doi.org/10.3390/healthcare14050630

Rivoli et al. (contribution 5) provide longitudinal evidence on changes in depressive symptoms and cognitive function in older adults, enriching the field's understanding of how mental health and cognition evolve over time in routine care populations—domains that are frequently implicated in fall vulnerability and post-fall recovery.

At the population level, Alves et al. (contribution 6) provide epidemiological evidence for Portugal using national emergency surveillance data, enhancing understanding of the frequency, distribution, and characteristics of fall-related unintentional injuries and supporting the identification of priority groups and injury patterns relevant to public health targeting and resource planning. Their findings indicate that falls among older adults increase with advancing age and occur predominantly in the settings where individuals spend most of their time, particularly the home. The study further suggests that prevention efforts should prioritise older women and focus on the domestic environment, with additional attention to higher-risk periods such as morning routines when daily activities may increase exposure to hazards.

Complementing this, Matos et al. (contribution 7) provide practice-relevant insight into older adults' perceptions of fall prevention and their engagement in social prescribing activities, strengthening understanding of acceptability, motivation, and participation—factors that shape whether evidence-based interventions are adopted and sustained beyond clinical settings. Their findings suggest that perceptions of fall prevention are embedded in broader patterns of engagement in health-promoting behaviours. Recognising and addressing differences in how older adults value and prioritise these activities can support the design of more inclusive, person-centred, and better targeted nursing interventions.

At the health-system performance level, Satoh et al. (contribution 8) extend the evidence base by evaluating risk-adjusted inpatient falls as safety indicators during the COVID-19 period, reinforcing the view that falls should be monitored not only as individual adverse events but also as system-level metrics responsive to organisational pressures and shifts in care delivery. Their findings suggest that risk-adjusted fall monitoring can detect dynamic changes in hospital safety performance during periods of major system strain and subsequent adaptation. Such indicators also have potential value for routine benchmarking, enabling month-to-month and seasonal safety surveillance beyond crisis contexts.

Finally, Ko et al. (contribution 9) add mechanistic insight by showing how fear of falling in people with low vision —experimentally modulated using virtual-reality simulation—can delay postural responses during gait initiation in people with low vision, strengthening the evidence that sensory impairment and fear-related motor control changes may compound fall risk and suggesting a pathway for targeted interventions that address both perceptual constraints and fear-driven movement strategies. Overall, these studies collectively advance fall knowledge by linking measurement to prevention, connecting clinical and psychosocial determinants, and situating falls within community, institutional, emergency, and system-performance contexts.

Overall, this Special Issue reinforces that meaningful progress in fall prevention will depend on integrating robust risk assessment with multifactorial, person-centred, and context-adapted interventions across the full continuum of care and diverse clinical practice settings.

5. Future Research Directions

One recommendation is that studies determining risk factors use a more comprehensive approach, exploring different domains—biophysiological, behavioural, environmental, and organisational—to understand the interaction between them. For the generation of comparable data, it is important to develop international recommendations on the risk factors to be collected in risk studies.

https://doi.org/10.3390/healthcare14050630

Another challenge for research is the evaluation of smart home innovations, interdisciplinary approaches, and the feasibility of policy implementation to support sustainable ageing-in-place strategies [30]. Digital health solutions (e.g., wearables and mobile apps) are promising for monitoring gait and activity and for supporting engagement, but they require validated endpoints, explicit attention to bias and equity (including digital exclusion), robust governance, integration into clinical workflows, and evidence of improvements in hard outcomes such as falls and injuries. Persistent heterogeneity in outcome definitions and measurement—including fall ascertainment methods, injurious falls, fear of falling, and functional outcomes—continues to limit evidence synthesis and guideline certainty. Moreover, many trials under-represent the oldest-old, minority ethnic groups, rural populations, and low- and middle-income settings, underscoring the need for culturally adapted interventions and cost-effectiveness evidence across diverse health systems.

Another comparatively underexplored area, requiring stronger evidence, is the development and evaluation of interventions that improve adherence to fall prevention education programmes—both sustained participation in prescribed, individualised physical activity and lasting adoption of safer everyday behaviours that reduce older adults' exposure to fall risk [32].

Fall prevention is still too often siloed from fracture prevention. Integrated pathways that reduce both falls and fall-related injuries, supported by stronger evidence for combined strategies (e.g., exercise alongside osteoporosis management and hip protectors for selected high-risk groups), remain a key priority. Increasingly, comprehensive care explicitly links falls and fracture prevention through osteoporosis assessment and treatment, ensuring adequate vitamin D and calcium when indicated, and considering hip protectors for selected high-risk residents.

Implementation research is still needed to determine how best to deliver programmes in routine services while maintaining intervention fidelity and quality, particularly in contexts of constrained staffing and funding, and how to support adherence over months to years.

There was a lack of studies addressing policy-level interventions and other relevant factors, such as environmental support. Moreover, the absence of long-term follow-up in many studies makes it difficult to assess the sustainability of the interventions [27].

6. Conclusions

In conclusion, fall prevention is not a "one-size-fits-all" intervention but a core pillar of geriatric nursing that depends on person-centred, evidence-informed assessment and coordinated action across settings. This Special Issue highlights that meaningful reductions in falls and fall-related harm come from combining clinical vigilance with system-level supports, early identification of multifactorial risk, medication and mobility review, safe environments, strength and balance promotion, appropriate use of assistive technology, and purposeful engagement of older adults and their caregivers in shared decision-making.

Taken together, the contributions reinforce that geriatric nurses are uniquely positioned to lead this work—translating evidence into daily practice, managing risk, and advancing equity by tailoring strategies to diverse needs and resources. As populations age and care grows more complex, sustained investment in nursing education, interdisciplinary partnerships, implementation science, and robust measurement of outcomes will be essential. The challenge is urgent, but the path is clear: when nurses, teams, and organisations align around proactive prevention, we can reduce avoidable harm, support independence, and improve quality of life for older adults.

https://doi.org/10.3390/healthcare14050630

Conflicts of Interest: The authors declare no conflicts of interest.

List of Contributions:

1. Hong, S.; Kim, J.-S.; Choi, Y.-A. Predictive Validity of the Johns Hopkins Fall Risk Assessment Tool for Older Patients in Stroke Rehabilitation. *Healthcare* **2024**, *12*, 791. https://doi.org/10.3390/healthcare12070791.
2. Simo-Tabue, N.; Letchimy, L.; Mounsamy, L.; Rinaldo, L.; Vainqueur, L.; Ntsama-Essomba, M.-J.; Mallet, G.; Boucaud-Maitre, D.; Tabue Teguo, M. Association between Polypharmacy and Hospitalization among Older Adults Admitted to Emergency Departments for Falls in Guadeloupe: A Retrospective Cohort Study. *Healthcare* **2024**, *12*, 1471. https://doi.org/10.3390/healthcare12151471.
3. Pereira, M.E.A.; Santos, G.d.S.; Almeida, C.R.d.; Nunes, K.C.S.; Silva, M.C.M.d.; José, H.; Sousa, L.; Vitorino, L.M. Association between Falls, Fear of Falling and Depressive Symptoms in Community-Dwelling Older Adults. *Healthcare* **2024**, *12*, 1638. https://doi.org/10.3390/healthcare12161638.
4. Miura, T.; Kanoya, Y. Fall Risk Assessment and Prevention Strategies in Nursing Homes: A Narrative Review. *Healthcare* **2025**, *13*, 357. https://doi.org/10.3390/healthcare13040357.
5. Rivoli, F.M.S.; Galhardo, A.P.G.M.; Lucchetti, G.; Esper, L.A.; Ribeiro, Y.L.; de Souza Santos, G.; José, H.; Sousa, L.; Low, G.; Vitorino, L.M. One-Year Changes in Depressive Symptoms and Cognitive Function Among Brazilian Older Adults Attending Primary Care. *Healthcare* **2025**, *13*, 807. https://doi.org/10.3390/healthcare13070807.
6. Alves, T.; Silva, S.; Braz, P.; Papadakaki, M.; Aniceto, C.; Mexia, R.; Matias-Dias, C. Epidemiology of Falls Among Older Adults in Portugal: Analysis of Unintentional Injuries Reported by a National Emergency Surveillance System. *Healthcare* **2025**, *13*, 1160. https://doi.org/10.3390/healthcare13101160.
7. Matos, C.; Baixinho, C.R.; Alarcão, V.; Henriques, M.A.; Ferreira, R.O.; Nascimento, T.; Arriaga, M.; Alves, T.; Nogueira, P.; Costa, A. Perceptions of Fall Prevention and Engagement in Social Prescribing Activities Among Older Adults: A Cross-Sectional Study in Portugal. *Healthcare* **2025**, *13*, 3209. https://doi.org/10.3390/healthcare13243209.
8. Satoh, M.; Nakahori, T.; Shimada, T. Risk-Adjusted Inpatient Falls as Indicators of Health System Performance During the COVID-19 Pandemic. *Healthcare* **2026**, *14*, 358. https://doi.org/10.3390/healthcare14030358.
9. Ko, M.; Gupta, P.K.; Brusola, G.; Chea, M.R.; Ahuja, P.; Chao, T.; Welsh, R.L. Delayed Postural Responses to Fear of Falling During Gait Initiation in Low Vision: Insights from Virtual-Reality-Based Fear Simulation. *Healthcare* **2026**, *14*, 400. https://doi.org/10.3390/healthcare14030400.

References

1. World Health Organization. *Strategies for Preventing and Managing Falls Across the Life-Course [Internet]*; WHO: Geneva, Switzerland, 2021. Available online: https://iris.who.int/bitstream/handle/10665/340962/9789240021914-eng.pdf (accessed on 17 December 2025).
2. Sampaio, F.; Nogueira, P.; Ascenção, R.; Henriques, A.; Costa, A. The epidemiology of falls in Portugal: An analysis of hospital admission data. *PLoS ONE* **2021**, *16*, e0261456. [CrossRef]
3. Baixinho, C.L.; Dixe, M.D.A.; Madeira, C.; Alves, S.; Henriques, M.A. Falls in institutionalized elderly with and without cognitive decline: A study of some factors. *Dement. Neuropsychol.* **2019**, *13*, 116–121. [CrossRef]
4. Matos, C.; Baixinho, C.R.; Alarcão, V.; Henriques, M.A.; Ferreira, R.O.; Nascimento, T.; Arriaga, M.; Alves, T.; Nogueira, P.; Costa, A. Perceptions of fall prevention and engagement in social prescribing activities among older adults: A cross-sectional study in Portugal. *Healthcare* **2025**, *13*, 3209. [CrossRef]
5. Montero-Odasso, M.; Van der Velde, N.; Martin, F.C.; Petrovic, M.; Tan, M.P.; Ryg, J.; Aguilar-Navarro, S.; Alexander, N.B.; Becker, C.; Blain, H.; et al. World guidelines for falls prevention and management for older adults: A global initiative. *Age Ageing* **2022**, *51*, afac205. [CrossRef] [PubMed]
6. Xu, Q.; Ou, X.; Li, J. The risk of falls among the aging population: A systematic review and meta-analysis. *Front. Public Health* **2022**, *10*, 902599. [CrossRef] [PubMed]
7. Saunders, S.; D'Amore, C.; Hao, Q.; El-Moneim, N.A.; Richardson, J.; Kuspinar, A.; Beauchamp, M. Risk factors for falls in community-dwelling older adults: An umbrella review. *J. Am. Med. Dir. Assoc.* **2025**, *26*, 105765. [CrossRef]

https://doi.org/10.3390/healthcare14050630

Li, Y.; Hou, L.; Zhao, H.; Xie, R.; Yi, Y.; Ding, X. Risk factors for falls among community-dwelling older adults: A systematic review and meta-analysis. *Front. Med.* **2023**, *9*, 1019094. [CrossRef]
Heinzmann, J.; Rossen, M.L.; Efthimiou, O.; Baumgartner, C.; Wertli, M.M.; Rodondi, N.; Aubert, C.E.; Liechti, F.D. Risk factors for falls among hospitalized medical patients: A systematic review and meta-analysis. *Arch. Phys. Med. Rehabil.* **2025**, *106*, 292–299. [CrossRef] [PubMed]
Yang, H.; Jiang, Y.; Yang, X.; Zhu, C.; Luo, L.; Hao, W. Assessment of risk factors for falls in hospitalized older adults: A meta-analysis. *Res. Gerontol. Nurs.* **2024**, *17*, 238–245. [CrossRef]
Mao, A.; Su, J.; Ren, M.; Chen, S.; Zhang, H. Risk prediction models for falls in hospitalized older patients: A systematic review and meta-analysis. *BMC Geriatr.* **2025**, *25*, 29. [CrossRef]
Dormosh, N.; van de Loo, B.; Heymans, M.W.; Schut, M.C.; Medlock, S.; van Schoor, N.M.; van der Velde, N.; Abu-Hanna, A. A systematic review of fall prediction models for community-dwelling older adults: Comparison between models based on research cohorts and models based on routinely collected data. *Age Ageing* **2024**, *53*, afae131. [CrossRef] [PubMed]
Zhao, G.; Zhang, Y.; Luo, J.; Tong, Y.; Sui, W. Prediction models for falls risk among inpatients: A systematic review and meta-analysis. *J. Adv. Nurs.* **2025**, *82*, 1973–1990. [CrossRef] [PubMed]
Morris, M.E.; Webster, K.; Jones, C.; Hill, A.M.; Haines, T.; McPhail, S.; Kiegaldie, D.; Slade, S.; Jazayeri, D.; Heng, H.; et al. Interventions to reduce falls in hospitals: A systematic review and meta-analysis. *Age Ageing* **2022**, *51*, afac077. [CrossRef] [PubMed]
Lee, D.; Tak, S.H.; Choi, H. A systematic review of fall prevention interventions in frail older adults. *Geriatr. Nurs.* **2025**, *62*, 236–244. [CrossRef]
Cameron, I.D.; Dyer, S.M.; Panagoda, C.E.; Murray, G.R.; Hill, K.D.; Cumming, R.G.; Kerse, N. Interventions for preventing falls in older people in care facilities and hospitals. *Cochrane Database Syst. Rev.* **2018**, *9*, CD005465. [CrossRef]
Spoon, D.; de Legé, T.; Oudshoorn, C.; van Dijk, M.; Ista, E. Implementation strategies of fall prevention interventions in hospitals: A systematic review. *BMJ Open Qual.* **2024**, *13*, e003006. [CrossRef]
Pillay, J.; Gaudet, L.A.; Saba, S.; Vandermeer, B.; Ashiq, A.R.; Wingert, A.; Hartling, L. Falls prevention interventions for community-dwelling older adults: Systematic review and meta-analysis of benefits, harms, and patient values and preferences. *Syst. Rev.* **2024**, *13*, 289. [CrossRef]
Sherrington, C.; Fairhall, N.J.; Wallbank, G.K.; Tiedemann, A.; Michaleff, Z.A.; Howard, K.; Clemson, L.; Hopewell, S.; Lamb, S.E. Exercise for preventing falls in older people living in the community. *Cochrane Database Syst. Rev.* **2019**, *1*, CD012424. [CrossRef]
Shafizadeh, M.; Parvinpour, S.; Ali, K. Effect of home-based exercise on falls in community-dwelling older adults: An umbrella review. *Sport Sci. Health* **2022**, *19*, 743–756. [CrossRef]
Naseri, C.; McPhail, S.M.; Morris, M.E.; Haines, T.P.; Etherton-Beer, C.; Shorr, R.; Flicker, L.; Bulsara, M.; Lee, D.A.; Francis-Coad, J.; et al. Tailored education increased capability and motivation for fall prevention in older people after hospitalization. *Front. Public Health* **2021**, *9*, 683723. [CrossRef]
22. Pilastri, F.B.; Lopez, J.F.; Boateng, E.N.; Marques, N.R. What to know about falls in older adults? Risk factors, predictors, and therapeutic interventions. *Int. J. Environ. Res. Public Health* **2025**, *22*, 1863. [CrossRef]
23. Buyle, M.; Jung, Y.; Pavlou, M.; Gonzalez, S.C.; Bamiou, D.E. The role of motivation factors in exergame interventions for fall prevention in older adults: A systematic review and meta-analysis. *Front. Neurol.* **2022**, *13*, 903673. [CrossRef] [PubMed]
24. Bindawas, S.M.; Vennu, V.; Almarwani, M.; Alsaleh, H.M.; Alsaad, S.M. Effectiveness of mobile health application-based interventions for fall prevention in community-dwelling older adults: A systematic review and meta-analysis of randomized controlled trials. *Sensors* **2026**, *26*, 864. [CrossRef]
25. Leite, M.M.; Silva, A.O.; Funghetto, S.S.; de Lima, L.R.; Mezavila Abdelmur, S.B.; Pinheiro, H.A.; de Souza Silva, C.M.; Dutra, M.T.; Stival, M.M. Home-based exercise and fall prevention in older adults: Development, validation and usability of the Mais Equilibrio mobile app. *JMIR Aging* **2025**, *8*, e80724. [CrossRef]
26. Drahota, A.; Udell, J.E.; Mackenzie, H.; Pugh, M.T. Psychological and educational interventions for preventing falls in older people living in the community. *Cochrane Database Syst. Rev.* **2024**, *10*, CD013480. [CrossRef] [PubMed]
27. Glangkarn, S.; Chejor, P.; Nonsa-Ard, R.; Wongprachum, K.; Khodseewong, S.; Bourneow, C.; Porock, D. Fall prevention interventions in community-dwelling older people with cognitive impairment: A systematic review. *JBI Evid. Implement.* **2026**, *24*, 183–201. [CrossRef] [PubMed]
28. Pierre-Lallemand, W.; Coughlin, V.; Brown-Tammaro, G.; Pierluissi, H.; Williams, W. Nursing-led targeted strategies for preventing falls in older adults. *Geriatr. Nurs.* **2025**, *62*, 297–299. [CrossRef] [PubMed]
29. Baixinho, C.R.S.L.; Dixe, M.D.A.C.R.; Henriques, M.A.P. Falls in long-term care institutions for elderly people: Protocol validation. *Rev. Bras. Enferm.* **2017**, *70*, 740–746. [CrossRef]
30. Cha, S.M. A systematic review of home modifications for aging in place in older adults. *Healthcare* **2025**, *13*, 752. [CrossRef]

https://doi.org/10.3390/healthcare14050630

31. Keall, M.D.; Tupara, H.; Pierse, N.; Wilkie, M.; Baker, M.G.; Howden-Chapman, P.; Cunningham, C. Home modifications prevent home fall injuries in houses with MƒÅori occupants (MHIPI): A randomized controlled trial. *Lancet Public Health* **2021** e631–e640. [CrossRef]
32. Palmer, S.J. Preventive measures for falls and fractures in the community. *Br. J. Community Nurs.* **2025**, *30*, 520–522. [CrossR [PubMed]

https://doi.org/10.3390/healthcare14050630

healthcare MDPI

icle

isk-Adjusted Inpatient Falls as Indicators of Health System erformance During the COVID-19 Pandemic

sae Satoh [1,*], Toko Nakahori [1] and Tomoko Shimada [2]

1 Department of Nursing, Graduate School of Medicine, Yokohama City University, 3-9 Fukuura, Kanazawa-ku, Yokohama 236-0004, Japan; t226612b@yokohama-cu.ac.jp
2 Nursing Department, Yokohama City University Hospital, Yokohama City University, 3-9 Fukuura, Kanazawa-ku, Yokohama 236-0004, Japan; s_tomoko@yokohama-cu.ac.jp
* Correspondence: m_satoh@yokohama-cu.ac.jp

Highlights

What are the main findings?

- Risk-adjusted inpatient fall indicators changed systematically during periods of monthly and large-scale system stress.
- Risk-adjusted safety performance improved over time despite increasing patient risk.

What are the implications of the main findings?

- Risk-adjusted fall monitoring supports the evaluation of hospital safety performance during seasonal changes and system-wide disruptions.
- Benchmarking fall outcomes provides a practical approach for safety surveillance in acute care settings.

Abstract

Background/Objectives: Inpatient falls are widely used patient safety indicators, yet their behavior under periods of large-scale health system stress remains insufficiently understood. This study aimed to evaluate whether risk-adjusted inpatient fall indicators can capture changes in hospital safety performance during such periods, using a prolonged system disruption as an empirical context. The study period was a priori divided into three phases (pre-pandemic, initial pandemic, and later pandemic) according to changes in COVID-19 admission burden and system stress intensity. **Methods:** We conducted a retrospective observational time-series analysis using daily inpatient fall events and census data from a Japanese acute care hospital between December 2018 and March 2023 (50,140 inpatients; 962 falls). Expected fall rates were estimated using a validated pre-disruption prediction model, and observed/expected (O/E) ratios were calculated to assess risk-adjusted safety performance. Ordinary least squares regression models adjusted for calendar month and seasonal Fourier terms were used to examine temporal associations between fall outcomes and indicators of hospital-level system burden. **Results:** Both observed and expected fall rates increased during the study period, whereas O/E ratios declined only in the later phase, indicating improvement in risk-adjusted safety performance despite rising intrinsic patient risk. Seasonal patterns in fall outcomes were disrupted during the early phase of system stress but re-emerged over time. Associations between system burden indicators and fall outcomes were most pronounced in the early phase and attenuated in later phases. **Conclusions:** Risk-adjusted monitoring of inpatient falls provides insight into dynamic changes in hospital safety performance during periods of large-scale system stress and subsequent adaptation. This indicator can also be interpreted as a benchmarking scale for future month-to-month and seasonal safety surveillance beyond crisis contexts.

Keywords: patient safety; inpatient falls; risk adjustment; benchmarking; health system performance; acute care; nursing; seasonality; system stress

1. Introduction

Inpatient falls are among the most common adverse events in acute care hospitals and are associated with fractures, loss of independence in activities of daily living, and prolonged hospitalization [1,2]. Because fall events are closely linked to nursing surveillance, care processes, and ward-level organization, inpatient fall rates are widely used as patient safety indicators in hospital quality monitoring [3,4].

Extensive research has focused on identifying patient-level risk factors for inpatient falls and developing predictive models to support targeted prevention strategies [5–7]. While these efforts have advanced individual risk stratification, they provide limited insight into how fall outcomes function as indicators of hospital-level safety performance over time.

Periods of large-scale system stress—such as the COVID-19 pandemic—can substantially alter staffing patterns, workflows, and care priorities in acute care settings [8–10]. During the COVID-19 pandemic, hospitals experienced marked fluctuations in patient volume, infection control demands, and staffing availability, all of which may have affected fall prevention practices. Although several studies have reported changes in fall incidence during the pandemic, most have relied on crude fall rates without accounting for underlying patient risk [11,12].

Risk-adjusted monitoring using observed-to-expected (O/E) ratios has been proposed as a more precise indicator of care quality and safety performance [13,14]. However, to date, no temporal analyses have examined the association between O/E ratios for inpatient falls and hospital-level COVID-19 burden. Moreover, since system-level exhaustion and operational disruptions may not manifest immediately, the potential time-lagged relationships between changes in COVID-19 admissions and subsequent variations in fall outcomes remain largely unexplored.

In Japan, patients with COVID-19 were first admitted to acute care hospitals in February 2020, followed by repeated declarations of a national state of emergency through September 2021, a period characterized by substantial strain on hospital systems and sustained changes in clinical operations [15,16]. After this period, social and healthcare practices gradually returned to pre-pandemic conditions.

Therefore, this study aimed to describe temporal changes in observed and expected fall rates—and in observed-to-expected (O/E) ratios—in general acute care wards during the COVID-19 pandemic and to assess their associations with new COVID-19 admissions using lag analysis. Expected fall rates were estimated using a pre-pandemic fall prediction model previously developed and validated in an acute care setting [17], allowing us to evaluate how hospital safety performance deviated from pre-pandemic standards.

2. Materials and Methods

2.1. Aim

This study aimed to evaluate longitudinal changes in inpatient fall outcomes using a risk-standardized benchmarking approach under COVID-19 burden. Specifically, the objectives were to (1) characterize temporal patterns in observed fall rates, expected fall rates, and O/E ratios across distinct phases of system disruption and (2) explore temporal associations between indicators of system burden and fall outcomes.

https://doi.org/10.3390/healthcare14030358

2.2. Design

This study employed a retrospective, observational time-series design, incorporating risk-standardized benchmarking, to evaluate inpatient safety performance under system-level stress. This study was reported in accordance with the Strengthening the Reporting of Observational Studies in Epidemiology (STROBE) guidelines.

2.3. Setting and Data

This study was conducted at a large acute care hospital in Japan using daily inpatient fall events and census data collected between 1 December 2018 and 31 March 2023. A 26-item fall risk assessment score routinely administered upon admission was used for baseline risk evaluation [17]. Fall events were obtained from the hospital's incident reporting system, and inpatient census data were extracted from administrative records. For analytical purposes, the study period was divided into three phases: a pre-pandemic period, an initial pandemic period during which national states of emergency were declared, and a later pandemic period without active emergency declarations. All analyses were conducted across these three periods, as illustrated in Figure 1.

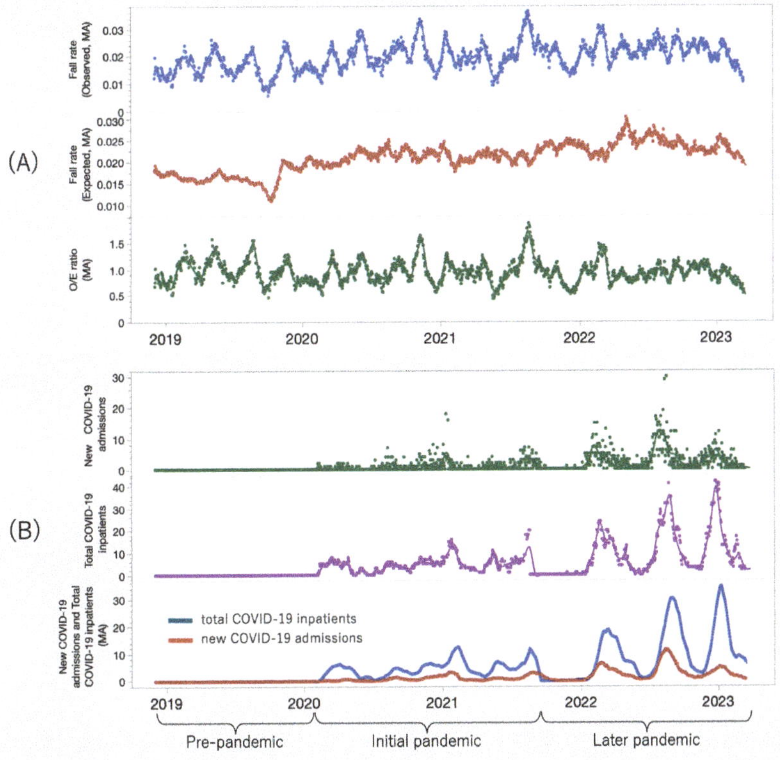

Figure 1. Temporal trends in fall-related outcomes and COVID-19 burden during the study period. (**A**) The 28-day moving averages of observed fall rates, expected fall rates, and observed-to-expected ratios. (**B**) Daily counts of new COVID-19 admissions and total COVID-19 inpatients, with respective 28-day moving averages. Time periods: pre-pandemic (1 December 2018–8 February 2020); initial pandemic (9 February 2020–30 September 2021); later pandemic (1 October 2021–31 March 2023).

Patients aged 16 years or older who were admitted to general wards and discharged during the study period were included. Patients admitted to intensive care, psychiatric, pe-

https://doi.org/10.3390/healthcare14030358

diatric, or designated infectious disease units were excluded. In total, 50,140 inpatients and 962 fall events met the inclusion criteria. To characterize system-level burden, daily counts of new COVID-19 admissions and the total number of hospitalized patients with COVID-19 were recorded as indicators of acute and sustained operational pressure, respectively.

2.4. Measures

The primary outcome was the observed fall rate, summarized using 28-day moving averages to reduce short-term variability. This window length was selected to provide a stable representation of temporal trends while preserving the interpretability of longitudinal changes.

Expected fall rates were estimated using a validated pre-pandemic logistic regression model [17]. The fixed six-factor model comprised the following binary predictors: age $\geq$65 years, impaired extremities, muscle weakness, requirement for mobility assistance, unstable gait, and psychotropic medication use. The model generated individual fall probabilities based on regression coefficients rather than a point-based scoring system.

The regression equation was specified as

$$\text{Logit}(p) = -3.048 + 0.339\,(\text{Age} \geq 65) + 0.340\,(\text{Impaired extremities}) + 0.492\,(\text{Muscle weakness}) + 0.418\,(\text{Mobility assistance}) + 0.466\,(\text{Unstable gait}) + 0.342\,(\text{Psychotropic medication use}),$$

where p denotes the probability of an inpatient fall, and $p = 1/[1 + \exp(-\text{Logit}(p))]$.

In the original validation cohort, the model demonstrated acceptable discriminative performance, with an area under the receiver operating characteristic curve of approximately 0.78. Model coefficients were not recalibrated during the pandemic period in order to preserve a fixed pre-disruption risk standard.

The O/E ratio, calculated as the observed fall rate divided by the expected fall rate, served as the primary risk-standardized indicator of safety performance, allowing deviations from unity to reflect changes in system-level safety performance rather than shifts in individual risk composition.

System burden was represented using two indicators: (1) the daily number of new COVID-19 admissions, reflecting acute system pressure, and (2) the total number of hospitalized patients with COVID-19, representing sustained operational burden. These indicators were used to contextualize safety performance under fluctuating care demands rather than as causal determinants of fall events.

2.5. Statistical Analysis

Ordinary least squares (OLS) time-series regression models were fitted separately for each phase of system disruption to examine associations between system burden indicators and fall outcomes. This phase-stratified approach enabled a direct comparison of association patterns under differing levels of system strain. Calendar-month fixed effects and Fourier seasonal terms were included to account for policy-related and cyclic variation.

OLS regression was selected to provide a transparent and interpretable framework for estimating average temporal associations, consistent with the study's descriptive and exploratory objectives rather than predictive forecasting. To mitigate short-term autocorrelation, fall-related outcomes and system burden indicators were smoothed using 28-day moving averages, and residual diagnostics were inspected to assess serial dependence.

Additional exploratory analyses using lagged indicators ranging from 0 to 28 days were conducted to support the interpretation of temporal patterns in fall outcomes. These lag analyses were theoretically motivated by the assumption that system strain may influence safety outcomes with a delayed effect due to cumulative disruptions in staffing and care processes. These analyses were not intended for causal inference.

Differences in regression coefficients across phases were interpreted as indicative of changes in the strength of association under varying system conditions rather than

https://doi.org/10.3390/healthcare14030358

as formal interaction effects. All statistical analyses were performed using JMP Student Edition version 18.2.0 (SAS Institute, Cary, NC, USA). A two-sided *p*-value of <0.05 was considered statistically significant.

2.6. Ethical Considerations

This study used routinely collected, de-identified data and was conducted in accordance with institutional and national ethical standards for research. This study was approved by the Ethics Committee of Epidemiological Research of Yokohama City University (approval number: F230800007; approval date: 15 September 2023). Study details were publicly disclosed on the hospital website to allow eligible individuals to opt out. All data were anonymized prior to analysis and securely stored on password-protected servers with restricted access.

3. Results

Overall, inpatient fall outcomes exhibited distinct temporal patterns across pandemic phases. While observed and expected fall rates increased over time, risk-adjusted O/E ratios showed phase-specific shifts, and associations with COVID-19 burden varied between the initial and later pandemic periods. These patterns are described below, beginning with descriptive trends followed by phase-specific regression results.

3.1. Temporal Patterns in Fall Indicators Across Pandemic Phases

Across the study period, observed fall rates showed greater short-term variability than expected fall rates, while O/E ratios remained centered around unity with phase-specific shifts.

Figure 1A depicts the 28-day moving averages of observed fall rates, expected fall rates, and O/E ratios. Observed fall rates exhibited pronounced short-term variability, particularly during the initial pandemic phase, whereas fluctuations stabilized in the later phase. Expected fall rates increased gradually and consistently throughout the study period. As expected from their construction, O/E ratios closely followed observed fall dynamics, although with a lower magnitude than raw incidence.

Table 1 presents least-squares means (±SEM) based on 28-day averaged data, adjusted for calendar month and pandemic phase. The mean observed fall rate increased from 1.63% in the pre-pandemic phase to 2.05% in the initial phase and 2.12% in the later phase. Expected fall rates demonstrated a similar upward trend (1.68%, 2.12%, and 2.36%, respectively). The O/E ratio remained near unity during the pre-pandemic (0.98) and initial (0.97) phases before declining to 0.90 in the later phase, indicating improved risk-adjusted safety performance despite rising intrinsic patient risk.

Table 1. Summary statistics of observed fall rates, expected fall rates, and O/E ratios across pandemic phases.

Variable	Pre-Pandemic	Initial Pandemic	Later Pandemic	Tukey–Kramer Test ($p < 0.05$)
Observed fall rate (%)	1.63 ± 0.02	2.05 ± 0.02	2.12 ± 0.02	Initial > Pre; Later > Pre
Expected fall rate (%)	1.68 ± 0.01	2.12 ± 0.01	2.36 ± 0.01	Initial > Pre; Later > Initial; Later > Pre
O/E ratio	0.98 ± 0.01	0.97 ± 0.01	0.90 ± 0.01	Later < Pre; Later < Initial

Values are expressed as least squares means ± standard errors derived from 28-day moving average (MA) data analyzed with general linear models, including fixed effects for period and month. Post hoc Tukey–Kramer HSD tests were applied for pairwise comparisons among periods. ">" and "<" indicate $p < 0.05$.

3.2. System Pressure Dynamics: COVID-19 Admission Patterns

COVID-19 system burden exhibited distinct short-term and cumulative dynamics over time.

https://doi.org/10.3390/healthcare14030358

Figure 1B depicts daily new COVID-19 admissions alongside the total number of hospitalized patients with COVID-19. Peaks in total inpatient census consistently followed surges in new admissions, reflecting the accumulation of system pressure over subsequent days rather than an immediate surge. This temporal pattern provides important context for interpreting subsequent safety outcomes.

3.3. Phase-Specific Regression Results: Seasonal and COVID-19-Related Effects

Associations between fall indicators and COVID-19 burden differed by pandemic phase and outcome type.

Figure 2 summarizes the ordinary least squares (OLS) regression estimates; full coefficient estimates are provided in Supplementary Table S1. Table 2 presents regression coefficients for COVID-19-related variables.

(A) Observed fall rate

(B) Expected fall rate

(C) O/E ratio

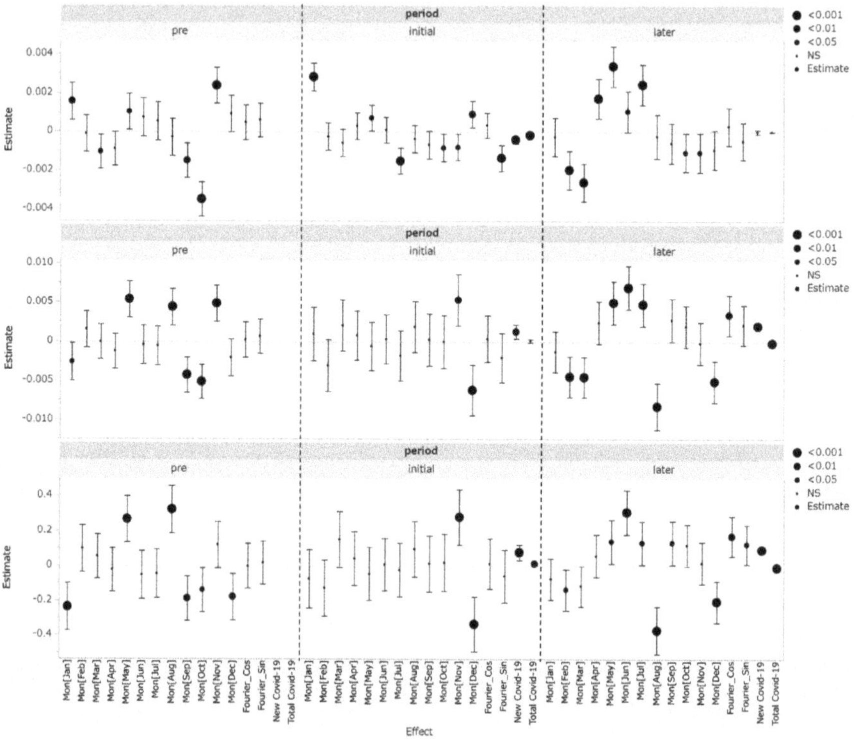

Figure 2. Monthly and COVID-19-related effects on fall rates and O/E ratios across pandemic phases. Estimates and 95% confidence intervals were sourced from ordinary least squares regression models, including month effects, Fourier terms, and COVID-19 related-variables. Significance levels are indicated by symbol size. New COVID-19 and Total COVID-19 represent new COVID-19 admissions and total COVID-19 inpatients, respectively.

Table 2. The linear regression results for fall outcomes by pandemic period (initial and later): the effects of COVID-19-related variables (simplified version).

Outcome	Effect	Initial		Later	
		Est (95% CI) *	p Value	Est (95% CI) *	p Value
Observed fall rate	Intercept	19.12 (18.35–19.88)	<0.001	17.64 (−17.05–18.23)	<0.001
	New COVID-19 admissions	1.28 (0.36–2.20)	<0.01	1.98 (1.71–2.26)	<0.001
	Total COVID-19 inpatients	0.09 (−0.11–0.29)	NS	−0.20 (−0.26–−0.14)	<0.001

https://doi.org/10.3390/healthcare14030358

Table 2. *Cont.*

Outcome	Effect	Initial		Later	
		Est (95% CI) *	*p* Value	Est (95% CI) *	*p* Value
Expected fall rate	Intercept	22.38 (22.21–22.54)	<0.001	23.76 (23.53–23.98)	<0.001
	New COVID-19 admissions	−0.39 (−0.58–−0.19)	<0.001	0.01 (−0.09–0.11)	NS
	Total COVID-19 inpatients	−0.16 (−0.20–−0.12)	<0.001	0.02 (−0.01–0.04)	NS
O/E ratio	Intercept	0.84 (0.81–0.88)	<0.001	0.72 (0.70–0.75)	<0.001
	New COVID-19 admissions	0.08 (0.03–0.12)	<0.001	0.09 (0.08–0.10)	<0.001
	Total COVID-19 inpatients	0.01 (0.00–0.02)	<0.01	−0.01 (−0.01–−0.01)	<0.001

Values are expressed as regression coefficients with 95% confidence intervals (CIs). Only COVID-19–related variables (new admissions and total inpatients) are shown. Full results, including month and seasonal terms, are provided in Supplementary Table S1. Lag analyses are reported separately in Supplementary Table S2. *: Estimates and 95% confidence interval limits for observed and expected fall rates are scaled ×1000 for clarity. Accordingly, regression coefficients should be interpreted as changes per 1000 units of the outcome.

3.3.1. Observed Fall Rate

Seasonal oscillations were pronounced during the pre-pandemic phase, as reflected by significant monthly peaks and troughs (Figure 2A). During the initial pandemic phase, these seasonal patterns largely disappeared, whereas new COVID-19 admissions were positively associated with observed fall rates, indicating heightened system strain during this phase. In the later phase, seasonal rhythms re-emerged, as evidenced by significant Fourier cosine terms, and the new COVID-19 burden remained positively associated with observed falls. In contrast, total COVID-19 inpatient counts showed an inverse association, suggesting potential changes in the system's response over time.

3.3.2. Expected Fall Rate

Expected fall rates demonstrated minimal seasonal fluctuation and no evident cyclic pattern (Figure 2B). During the initial pandemic phase, both new COVID-19 admissions and total COVID-19 inpatient counts were negatively associated with expected fall rates. In the later phase, no significant associations were observed, indicating that the patient case mix stabilized over time.

3.3.3. Observed-to-Expected (O/E) Ratio

The O/E ratio closely mirrored the temporal patterns of observed fall rates, which is consistent with the relative stability of expected rates (Figure 2C). Seasonal effects were attenuated during the initial phase but re-emerged in the later phase, as indicated by significant Fourier sine and cosine terms. New COVID-19 admissions were consistently and positively associated with O/E ratios across all phases. In contrast, total COVID-19 inpatient counts shifted from a positive association in the initial phase to a significant negative association in the later phase, indicating a shift in the association between system burden and risk-adjusted fall outcomes over time.

3.4. *Exploratory Temporal Associations Between Fall Rates and COVID-19 Burden*

Time-lagged associations between new COVID-19 admissions and observed fall rates varied across pandemic phases.

Figure 3 shows exploratory temporal associations between new COVID-19 admissions and inpatient fall rates across lag intervals ranging from 0 to 28 days. During the initial pandemic phase, positive associations were observed consistently across all examined lag intervals, whereas during the later phase, these associations were attenuated and less consistent across lag structures. These analyses were conducted to aid the interpretation of temporal patterns in fall outcomes. Full regression results are provided in Supplementary Table S2.

https://doi.org/10.3390/healthcare14030358

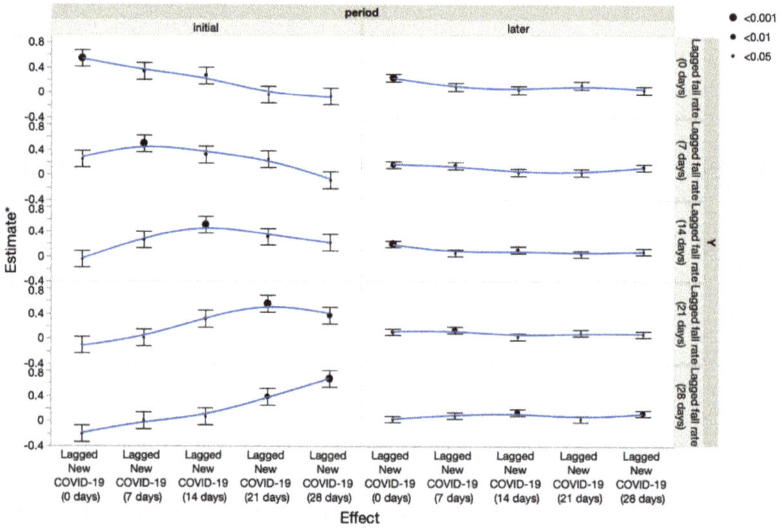

Figure 3. Synchronized temporal associations between fall rates and new COVID-19 admissions across lag intervals (0, 7, 14, 21, and 28 days), stratified by pandemic phase (initial and later). Estimates ± standard errors from lag-specific regression models are plotted for each phase, with significance levels represented by dot size and trends connected by smoothed lines. Associations were stronger and showed clearer lag-dependent patterns in the initial phase, but weakened and became less consistent in the later phase. *: Estimates are scaled ×1000 for clarity.

4. Discussion

This study examined longitudinal changes in inpatient fall outcomes during periods of large-scale system stress using a risk-adjusted benchmarking approach. Directly supported by our data, observed and expected fall rates increased during the pandemic, whereas the observed-to-expected (O/E) ratio declined only in the later phase. This pattern indicates that changes in crude fall rates and changes in risk-adjusted safety performance did not occur in parallel, underscoring the value of risk-adjusted surveillance for disentangling shifts in patient case mix from changes in system-level performance.

Previous studies conducted during the COVID-19 pandemic primarily reported higher inpatient fall rates based on crude incidence measures, which limit the interpretation of hospital safety performance under disrupted care conditions [11,12]. In contrast, our findings show that risk-adjusted indicators can capture phase-specific changes in safety performance that are not apparent from crude rates alone. This observation suggests that exclusive reliance on unadjusted fall rates may obscure important aspects of organizational performance during prolonged periods of system disruption.

Before the pandemic, inpatient fall outcomes demonstrated regular seasonal variations, consistent with prior research on hospital safety rhythms. Our descriptive and regression analyses indicate that these seasonal patterns were attenuated during the initial phase of the pandemic. Similar disruption of routine safety processes has been reported during early phases of large-scale healthcare emergencies [9,18]. An interpretation consistent with these observations is that acute system stress may temporarily disrupt established organizational rhythms related to patient safety.

Differences observed across pandemic phases likely reflect varying degrees of system strain over time. In Japan, the early pandemic period was marked by repeated emergency declarations and rapid organizational reconfiguration, including the admission of patients

https://doi.org/10.3390/healthcare14030358

from the Diamond Princess cruise ship, which imposed substantial psychological and operational stress on healthcare staff [15,16]. Subsequent studies have suggested that such strain may persist beyond the initial crisis phase [8,10,19]. In contrast, later phases coincided with partial organizational adaptation and stabilization of care delivery under sustained pressure [20]. These contextual factors provide a plausible backdrop for interpreting phase-specific patterns in fall indicators, although causal mechanisms cannot be established from the present observational data.

In later phases, seasonal regularity in fall outcomes re-emerged. While this pattern cannot be directly attributed to specific organizational changes, it is consistent with partial stabilization of hospital operations over time. Similarly, the shift in associations between total COVID-19 inpatient burden and fall outcomes across phases may reflect evolving care organization or staff responses under sustained system pressure. These interpretations should be regarded as hypothesis-generating rather than confirmatory.

Exploratory temporal analyses further showed that associations between system burden indicators and fall outcomes were strongest during the initial phase and attenuated in later phases. These findings are consistent with the hypothesis that safety outcomes may be more tightly coupled to operational strain during periods of acute disruption, with weaker coupling as systems adapt. Comparable time-dependent associations between external stressors and health outcomes have been described in other contexts, such as delayed health effects following environmental exposures or extreme events [21,22]. In the present study, lag analyses were intended to support the interpretation of temporal patterns rather than to infer causal relationships.

Inpatient falls are widely recognized as nursing-sensitive safety indicators influenced by patient characteristics, care processes, and ward-level conditions [23]. Taken together, our findings indicate that risk-adjusted inpatient fall indicators may be useful for monitoring hospital safety performance under fluctuating care demands. From an organizational and clinical governance perspective, such indicators may support nursing leaders and hospital safety teams in interpreting safety trends during periods of systemic stress, including workforce shortages or seasonal demand surges, beyond pandemic contexts.

5. Limitations

This study has several limitations. First, the fall prediction model used to estimate expected rates was calibrated using pre-pandemic data and did not incorporate disruption-specific care factors; therefore, changes in care environments during the pandemic may not have been fully captured. Second, this single-center study conducted in a Japanese acute care hospital may reflect context-specific organizational characteristics, limiting generalizability to other healthcare settings. Third, the observational design and temporal analyses examined associations rather than causal relationships, and the absence of detailed operational and staffing data precluded examination of underlying mechanisms. Future multicenter studies incorporating higher-resolution operational data are needed to further refine risk-adjusted safety monitoring approaches.

6. Conclusions

This study examined temporal patterns in inpatient fall outcomes during periods of large-scale system stress using a risk-adjusted benchmarking approach. The findings suggest that incorporating O/E ratios can support the interpretation of inpatient fall trends by accounting for concurrent changes in patient risk profiles and care environments. In this cohort, although both observed and expected fall rates increased during the pandemic, declines in O/E ratios were observed in later phases, indicating phase-specific variation in risk-adjusted fall outcomes that was not fully captured by crude fall rates alone.

https://doi.org/10.3390/healthcare14030358

By applying a risk-standardized approach to a nursing-sensitive safety indicator, this study highlights the potential value of distinguishing intrinsic patient risk from system-level influences when evaluating inpatient safety. Rather than serving as an exhaustive indicator of overall health system performance, the O/E ratio may function as a complementary tool to support safety monitoring and assessment, particularly during periods of disrupted or fluctuating care demand.

Taken together, these findings indicate that risk-adjusted inpatient fall indicators may assist nursing leaders and hospital safety teams in more accurately contextualizing safety performance under conditions of systemic stress, such as pandemics or workforce disruptions. Further multicenter research is required to evaluate the generalizability of this approach and to clarify how risk-adjusted indicators can be integrated into broader hospital safety surveillance and clinical governance frameworks.

Supplementary Materials: The following supporting information can be downloaded at: https://www.mdpi.com/article/10.3390/healthcare14030358/s1, Table S1: Linear regression results for fall outcomes by pandemic period (Pre, Initial, Later): Full model including month and seasonal terms; Table S2: Exploratory regression results for temporal associations between inpatient fall rates and new COVID-19 admissions across lag intervals (0–28 days).

Author Contributions: M.S.: Writing—review and editing, writing—original draft, visualization, validation, supervision, resources, project administration, methodology, investigation, funding acquisition, formal analysis, data curation, and conceptualization. T.N.: Writing—review and editing, validation, investigation, formal analysis, data curation, and conceptualization. T.S.: Writing—review and editing, investigation, formal analysis, data curation, and conceptualization. All authors have read and agreed to the published version of the manuscript.

Funding: This work was supported by the Japan Society for the Promotion of Science (JSPS) KAKENHI Grant-in-Aid for Scientific Research (B) Grant Number JP22H03377.

Institutional Review Board Statement: This retrospective observational study used routinely collected, de-identified data. The study was conducted in accordance with the Declaration of Helsinki, and approved by the Institutional Review Board of [Yokohama City University], Kanagawa, Japan (Approval No. F230800007, 15 September 2023). Study details were publicly disclosed on the hospital website to allow eligible individuals to opt out. The requirement for informed consent was waived due to the use of anonymized clinical data.

Informed Consent Statement: Informed consent was waived for this retrospective analysis.

Data Availability Statement: The datasets presented in this article are not readily available because the data are part of an ongoing study. Requests to access the datasets should be directed to the corresponding author.

Acknowledgments: The authors would like to thank Teppei Nishii of the Department of Medical Informatics at the university hospital for providing the data used in this study, Hideaki Kato of the Department of Infection Control for his guidance and support throughout the research process, and Tetsutaro Hamano for his valuable contributions to the statistical analysis and for reviewing the accuracy and interpretation of the results.

Conflicts of Interest: The authors declare no conflicts of interest.

Abbreviations

The following abbreviations are used in this manuscript:

COVID-19	Coronavirus disease 2019
O/E	Observed-to-expected
OLS	Ordinary least squares

https://doi.org/10.3390/healthcare14030358

ferences

LeLaurin, J.H.; Shorr, R.I. Preventing falls in hospitalized patients: State of the science. *Clin. Geriatr. Med.* **2019**, *35*, 273–283. [CrossRef]

Locklear, T.; Kontos, J.; Callaham, B.A. Inpatient falls: Epidemiology, risk assessment, and prevention measures—A narrative review. *HCA Healthc. J. Med.* **2024**, *5*, 7. [CrossRef]

Metersky, M.L.; Rodrick, D.; Ho, S.-Y.; Galusha, D.; Timashenka, A.; Grace, E.N.; Marshall, D.; Eckenrode, S.; Krumholz, H.M. Hospital COVID-19 burden and adverse event rates. *JAMA Netw. Open* **2024**, *7*, e2442936. [CrossRef]

Vincent, C.; Amalberti, R. *Safer Healthcare: Strategies for the Real World*; Springer: Cham, Switzerland, 2016. [CrossRef]

Hitcho, E.B.; Krauss, M.J.; Birge, S.; Dunagan, W.C.; Fischer, I.; Johnson, S.; Nast, P.A.; Costantinou, E.; Fraser, V.J. Characteristics and circumstances of falls in a hospital setting. *J. Gen. Intern. Med.* **2004**, *19*, 732–739. [CrossRef]

Oliver, D.; Healey, F.; Haines, T.P. Preventing falls and fall-related injuries in hospitals. *Clin. Geriatr. Med.* **2010**, *26*, 645–692. [CrossRef] [PubMed]

Nakanishi, T.; Ikeda, T.; Nakamura, T.; Yamanouchi, Y.; Chikamoto, A.; Usuku, K. Development of an algorithm for assessing fall risk in a Japanese inpatient population. *Sci. Rep.* **2021**, *11*, 17993. [CrossRef] [PubMed]

Couper, K.; Murrells, T.; Sanders, J.; Anderson, J.E.; Blake, H.; Kelly, D.; Kent, B.; Maben, J.; Rafferty, A.M.; Taylor, R.M.; et al. The impact of COVID-19 on the wellbeing of the UK nursing and midwifery workforce during the first pandemic wave. *Int. J. Nurs. Stud.* **2022**, *127*, 104155. [CrossRef]

Maben, J.; Conolly, A.; Abrams, R.; Rowland, E.; Harris, R.; Kelly, D.; Kent, B.; Couper, K. 'You can't walk through water without getting wet' UK nurses' distress during the COVID-19 pandemic. *Int. J. Nurs. Stud.* **2022**, *131*, 104242. [CrossRef]

Dragioti, E.; Tsartsalis, D.; Mentis, M.; Mantzoukas, S.; Gouva, M. Impact of the COVID-19 pandemic on the mental health of hospital staff: An umbrella review. *Int. J. Nurs. Stud.* **2022**, *131*, 104272. [CrossRef]

Liang, S.C.; Wei, P.C.; Ma, H.L.; Hsiao, S.H. Higher fall rate of admitted patients during COVID-19. *J. Patient Saf.* **2021**, *17*, e45–e46. [CrossRef] [PubMed]

. Shennan, S.; Coyle, N.; Lockwood, B.; DiDiodato, G. Visitor restrictions and increased falls with harm. *J. Patient Saf.* **2024**, *20*, 434–439. [CrossRef]

. Bernet, N.S.; Everink, I.H.J.; Schols, J.M.G.; Halfens, R.J.G.; Richter, D.; Hahn, S. Hospital performance comparison of inpatient fall rates. *BMC Health Serv. Res.* **2022**, *22*, 225. [CrossRef]

. Bernet, N.S.; Ros, A.; Rüesch, P.; Schwendimann, R.; Simon, M. Risk-adjusted trend in national inpatient fall rates. *BMJ Open* **2024**, *14*, e082417. [CrossRef]

. Ide, K.; Asami, T.; Suda, A.; Yoshimi, A.; Fujita, J.; Nomoto, M.; Roppongi, T.; Hino, K.; Takahashi, Y.; Watanabe, K.; et al. The Psychological effects of COVID-19 on hospital workers. *PLoS ONE* **2021**, *16*, e0245294. [CrossRef]

ː. Karako, K.; Song, P.; Chen, Y.; Karako, T. COVID-19 in Japan during 2020–2022. *J. Glob. Health* **2022**, *12*, 03073. [CrossRef] [PubMed]

'. Satoh, M.; Miura, T.; Shimada, T. Development and evaluation of a simple predictive model for falls. *J. Clin. Nurs.* **2023**, *32*, 6474–6484. [CrossRef]

3. Hartley, H.; Dunning, A.; Dunn, M.; Grange, A.; Murray, J.; Simms-Ellis, R.; Unsworth, K.; Marran, J.; Lawton, R. Managing nurse redeployment during COVID-19. *Int. J. Nurs. Stud.* **2024**, *157*, 104828. [CrossRef]

9. Ide, K.; Asami, T.; Suda, A.; Yoshimi, A.; Fujita, J.; Shiraishi, Y.; Nomoto, M.; Miyauchi, M.; Roppongi, T.; Furuno, T.; et al. The Psychological distress in hospital workers during COVID-19. *PLoS ONE* **2022**, *17*, e0277174. [CrossRef]

0. Adelman, J.S.; Gandhi, T.K. COVID-19 and patient safety: Time to tap into high reliability. *J. Patient Saf.* **2021**, *17*, 331–333. [CrossRef]

1. Huang, J.; Wang, J.; Yu, W. Lag effects of temperature on cardiovascular mortality. *Int. J. Environ. Res. Public Health* **2014**, *11*, 3982–3994. [CrossRef] [PubMed]

2. Peng, J.; Wu, X.; Chen, J.; Qian, J.; Li, N.; Yi, Y.; Huang, Y.; Lu, J.; Zhang, W.; Li, Z.; et al. Short-term effects of ambient air pollutants and meteorological factors on emergency department visits in tropical Haikou, China. *Sci. Rep.* **2025**, *15*, 7056. [CrossRef] [PubMed]

3. Takase, M. Falls as the result of interplay between nurses, patients and the environment. *Int. J. Nurs. Sci.* **2023**, *10*, 30–37. [CrossRef] [PubMed]

https://doi.org/10.3390/healthcare14030358

healthcare

MDPI

Article

Delayed Postural Responses to Fear of Falling During Gait Initiation in Low Vision: Insights from Virtual-Reality-Based Fear Simulation

Mansoo Ko [1,*], Praveena K. Gupta [2], Gregory Brusola [1], Metha R. Chea [2], Pranati Ahuja [2], Tony Chao [1] and Rodney L. Welsh [1]

[1] Department of Physical Therapy, School of Health Professions, University of Texas Medical Branch at Galveston, Galveston, TX 77555-1144, USA; gabrusol@utmb.edu (G.B.); tochao@utmb.edu (T.C.); rlwelsh@utmb.edu (R.L.W.)

[2] Department of Ophthalmology and Visual Sciences, School of Medicine, University of Texas Medical Branch at Galveston, Galveston, TX 77555-1144, USA; prgupta@utmb.edu (P.K.G.); mrchea@utmb.edu (M.R.C.)

[*] Correspondence: mako@utmb.edu

Abstract

Purpose: This study aimed to quantify the severity of fear of falling (FOF) in people with low vision (LV) compared with age–gender-matched healthy individuals during gait initiation (GI). **Methods:** A total of 14 adults with LV and 14 age–gender-matched healthy adults were recruited from local communities. The Falls Efficacy Scale International was used to evaluate FOF. We compared temporal events between healthy and LV groups. For the healthy group, GI under normal vision was further compared to conditions using a low-vision sight simulator (SS) and an immersive virtual reality (VR) environment designed to simulate a fear-evoking experience. Independent *t*-test and one-way repeated measure ANOVA were conducted for statistical analysis ($p < 0.05$). **Results:** People with LV showed a significantly greater FOF than healthy individuals ($p < 0.05$). During GI, participants with LV exhibited significantly prolonged anticipatory postural adjustment (APA) durations compared to healthy normal and SS conditions ($p < 0.05$). While VR-evoked fear in healthy participants primarily prolonged the push-off (PO) phase, the delay in the LV group was characterized by a significantly extended initial anticipation (AP) phase. Notably, the APA duration in the LV group showed no significant difference compared to the healthy VR condition, indicating that the inherent fear in LV produces postural delays as severe as those induced by extreme VR-evoked fear of heights ($p > 0.05$). **Conclusions:** This study demonstrates that individuals with LV adopt a chronically conservative motor program during the transition from standing to walking. These postural hesitations are statistically comparable to those observed under fear-evoking, VR-induced environments. These findings suggest that LV is associated with a distinct biomechanical strategy that prioritizes static stability over dynamic movement. Accordingly, multidisciplinary rehabilitation approaches that emphasize sensory reweighting, including vestibular training, alongside interventions targeting FOF, may be essential for mitigating altered postural control and reducing fall risk in the LV population.

Keywords: fear of falling; gait initiation; virtual reality; low vision; postural control

1. Introduction

Visual impairment (VI) is a primary cause of loss of independence among older adults. Globally, over 2.2 billion people live with VI, resulting in substantial annual costs for long-term services [1]. The total annual economic impact of vision loss and blindness in the United States reaches approximately $134.2 billion [2]. Specifically, fear of falling (FOF) is a major health concern for older adults with VI, often leading to complications such as falls, hip fractures, anxiety, depression, immobility, and functional dependence [3,4]. An estimated 48.3% of older adults with VI report FOF due to poor visual acuity, reduced contrast sensitivity, and loss of depth perception [5,6]. This fear significantly impacts anticipatory postural control, the process by which individuals adjust their postural balance or prepare to move prior to executing the first step from a standing position. Consequently, this FOF often triggers protective strategies such as stiffening the body, hesitating before initiating movement, or delaying actions, serving as preventive measures against potential falls [7]. Of equal concern is the contribution of FOF to fear-related activity and participation restriction in people with VI, with significant implications on their overall functional mobility [1,5,8].

Gait initiation (GI) is defined as a transitional period between quiet standing and the initiation of steady state walking. This common motor task is performed throughout the day by ambulatory individuals and is used to assess balance control during gait [9]. In regular walking patterns, GI includes both double and single support phases. It involves anticipatory postural adjustment (APA) to counteract the destabilizing postural balance caused by a rapid backward weight shift. Individuals with balance deficits often show reluctance to disrupt their static balance by delaying weight shifting during GI [9]. This delay in GI has been associated with the increased risk of multiple falls [10] and has recently been found to be strongly associated with increased reliance on vision in older adults [11]. Accordingly, the task of GI may maximize FOF-related control strategies to execute the first step by breaking the static balance in older adults with low vision (LV). Vision is critical for planning goal-directed movements because it defines the kinematic plan and modulates the scaling of movement prior to movement initiation [11,12]. Previous studies have shown that postural threat, such as exposure to elevated surfaces or virtual height environments, attenuates anticipatory postural adjustments and constrains weight shifting during gait initiation (GI) in healthy adults [13]. However, it remains unclear how fear disrupts movement control strategies during GI in individuals with LV. To address this gap, experimental paradigms that can systematically manipulate fear-related contextual factors during gait are essential. Traditional approaches to simulate visual impairment include optical blur lenses and prism-based visual perturbations [14,15]; however, these methods primarily alter sensory input and are limited in their ability to dynamically manipulate environmental threat and fear-related contextual factors during walking tasks [16]. Compounding these sensory constraints, conventional experimental paradigms frequently rely on highly repetitive tasks, which can reduce participant engagement and compromise sustained attention, particularly in frail older adults and clinical population. To address these limitations, virtual reality (VR)-based locomotion paradigms incorporate interactive and goal-directed tasks, such as collecting virtual targets via a full-body embodied avatar, to enhance motivation and mitigate the inherent monotony of gait-related protocols [17]. Beyond improving engagement, this approach enables the extraction of sensitive, trajectory-based metrics, including Normalized Path Length and Initial Angle Error, which provide quantitative measures of visuomotor adaptation and motor control performance [17]. Such high-fidelity data collection is particularly valuable in clinical settings for establishing recovery benchmarks and tailoring interventions for populations with neuromotor disorders.

Given that FOF is a multifactorial construct bridging physical instability and psychological apprehension, VR offers the unique advantage of systematically isolating and manipulating fear-related variables within a controlled, yet safe, environment [18,19]. VR-based technology allows for the simulation of visual input related to poor visual acuity,

https://doi.org/10.3390/healthcare14030400

reduced contrast sensitivity, loss of depth perception, and vertigo, leading to FOF. Importantly, simulating visual impairment in healthy individuals facilitates the acquisition of larger, more standardized datasets than are typically feasible with visually impaired populations. This approach is particularly valuable because data collection from individuals with actual visual or neuromotor impairments is often constrained by substantial practical and safety-related limitations. Due to physical fatigue, balance instability, and fall risk, pathological populations typically tolerate only a limited number of task repetitions and require longer rest periods between trials. Sample sizes are therefore frequently restricted, particularly in individuals with non-autonomous gait execution, and experimental sessions commonly necessitate continuous physician or clinical staff supervision to ensure participant safety. These constraints can substantially limit the volume, variability, and standardization of gait data that can be acquired from clinical populations. Recent work has highlighted these challenges and emphasized that simulating pathological gait or sensory impairments in healthy participants, when conducted under appropriate clinical guidance, provides a principled methodological strategy for acquiring larger and more standardized datasets prior to validation in clinical populations [20]. By enabling a greater number of repetitions under controlled conditions, this approach directly addresses the structural limitations inherent to clinical data acquisition and establishes a clear methodological rationale for the proposed workflow, while maintaining the safety and feasibility required for clinical research.

Consequently, this methodological framework mitigates common experimental constraints, such as limited task repetition and the extended recovery periods required by clinical participants due to fatigue and safety considerations. Previous studies have attempted to simulate VI in healthy individuals [21–23], but limited research exists on simulating and assessing FOF. It is still unknown whether the anxiety perceptions experienced in real environments mirror those in virtual contexts, especially when compared to individuals with VI [23]. To date, FOF is typically screened by clinical interviews or self-report instruments, which mainly rely on an individual's perception and memory and may lead to experiential bias. Thus, we propose that GI using VR technology could provide objective performance-based measures to quantify postural control due to FOF. This virtually simulated impairment in both healthy individuals and those with VI allows the examination of postural control strategies and their efficacy when transferring from standing to the first step of ambulation. Combining VR simulation with a balance measure device is a novel approach to identify balance deficits for individuals with a FOF and VI.

Therefore, the purpose of this study was to quantify the severity of FOF in people with LV compared to age- and gender-matched healthy individuals without LV. We hypothesized that individuals with LV would show a greater fear compared to healthy individuals and that the postural control strategies of people with LV during GI would be similar to those of people without LV when exposed to an immersive VR simulating FOF.

2. Methods

The systematic framework of this study, encompassing participant pre-task assessment, experimental design, data analysis and processing, and statistical evaluation is summarized in the proposed research pipeline.

2.1. Participants

Fourteen adults with LV (mean age 62 ± 15 years) were recruited via consecutive sampling from UTMB Health Eye Center-Galveston through referral by Doctor of Optometry, and 14 age–gender-matched adults without LV (mean age 63 ± 10 years) were recruited from local communities. A total of 33 participants were initially assessed for

https://doi.org/10.3390/healthcare14030400

eligibility; however, four healthy participants were excluded from the final analysis due to height-related VR fear, and two participants with low vision were unable to successfully complete the gait initiation task (Figure 1). Inclusion criteria for participants with LV included: being aged 18 years or older; having a diagnosis of VI confirmed through an eye examination within the last two years; reported fall within the last 24 months; capable of independent mobility, covering a minimum of 10 m without an assistive device at a comfortable speed; and able to understand the study's procedures, consent form, and follow the study team's instructions. Participants with a history of epilepsy, orthopedic, psychiatric, neurological, or cognitive impairments, as well as a history of substance abuse or who were currently pregnant were excluded. Low vision was defined as having a visual acuity of 20/70 or worse in the better-seeing eye or a constricted visual field of 20° or less. Ophthalmologists conducted eye examinations to ensure the credibility of participants with LV. Participants with LV represented a clinically heterogeneous group, ranging from moderate visual impairment to severe blindness, with variability in both visual acuity and visual field loss (Table 1). This heterogeneity reflects the real-world population of individuals with LV who experience balance challenges and fall risks, which may influence postural control strategies. The inclusion and exclusion criteria for participants without LV were the same except for the absence of VI, confirmed through a recent eye examination within the last two years. This study was approved by the Institutional Review Board of the University of Texas Medical Branch (UTMB IRB #21-016). All procedures were conducted in accordance with the Declaration of Helsinki, and written informed consent was obtained from all participants prior to participation.

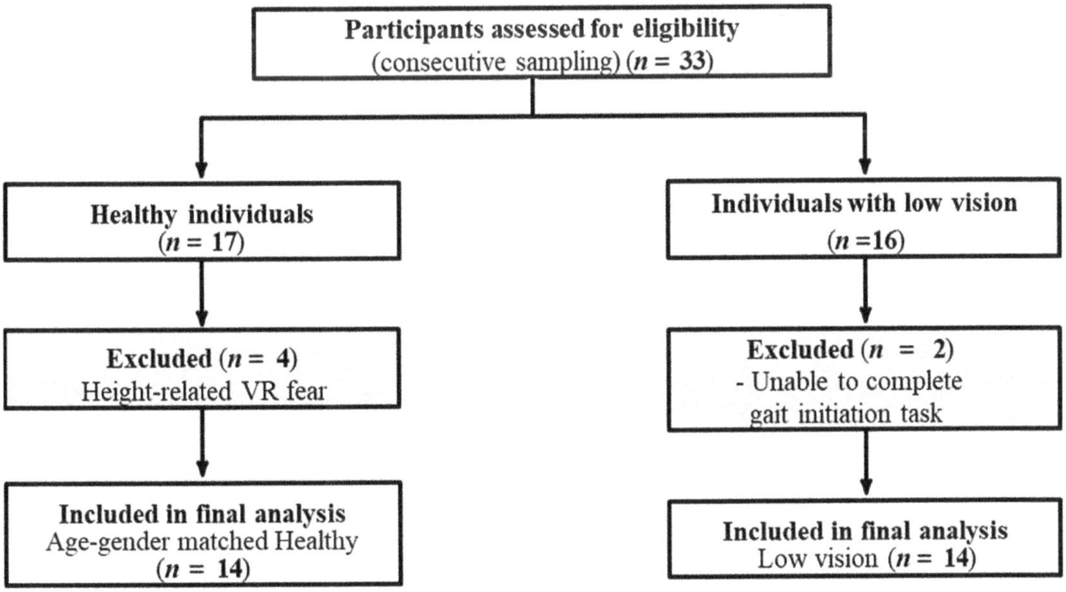

Figure 1. Participant flow diagram.

https://doi.org/10.3390/healthcare14030400

Table 1. Demographic information of participants with low vision.

Low Vision Subject	Gender	Age	Height (cm)	Weight (kg)	BMI	VA OD	VA OS	Visual Impairment Classification	FES-I
1	Female	50	163	62	24	20/400	20/125	Moderate Visual Impairment	34
2	Male	45	192	117	32	20/400	20/400	Blindness	45
3	Female	79	160	73	29	CF at 3ft	CF at 3ft	Severe Blindness	44
4	Male	70	178	115	36	20/150	20/150	Moderate Visual Impairment	22
5	Female	67	152	76	33	20/300	20/300	Blindness	46
6	Female	66	168	83	29	20/200	20/400	Moderate Visual Impairment	19
7	Female	70	173	100	34	20/400	CF at 3ft	Blindness	39
8	Male	59	168	83	30	20/400	NLP	Blindness	36
9	Male	87	157	76	31	20/400	CF at 1ft	Blindness	44
10	Female	68	152	62	27	20/400	20/100	Moderate Visual Impairment	55
11	Male	26	173	80	27	CF at 3ft	CF at 3ft	Severe Blindness	23
12	Male	75	170	72	25	20/200	20/200	Moderate Visual Impairment	18
13	Male	50	168	80	29	20/80	CF at 3ft	Moderate Visual Impairment	31
14	Female	55	168	97	34	20/70 * Constricted VF 10 degrees	20/20	Severe blindness	64
Mean ± SD		62 ± 15	167 ± 11	84 ± 17	30 ± 4				37 ± 14

* Severe blindness was classified based on a constricted visual field of 10 degrees rather than visual acuity. Abbreviations: VA: Visual acuity, OD: Oculus dexter (right eye), OS: Oculus sinister (left eye), CF: Count Finger, VF: Visual field, FES-I: Falls Efficacy Scale International.

2.2. Procedures

All data collection procedures were conducted by trained clinicians with experience in gait initiation and balance assessment. Prior to the task of GI, participants were assessed using the Falls Efficacy Scale International (FES-I). The 16-item FES-I was developed as a modification of the original Falls Efficacy Scale (FES) as a suitable measure to use across language and cultural contexts in the assessment of FOF [24]. While the FES assesses confidence, the FES-I measures the concern of an individual in performing a range of daily activities without falling, including activities such as transitional movements, stair negotiation, walking outside, and engaging in social activities [24]. The FES-I total score ranges from 16 to 64 with higher scores indicating greater FOF [25]. The FES-I has been found to be valid and reliable in assessing fear of falling [26–28] and has been used previously in individuals with visual impairment [29–32]. Following the assessment of the FES-I, both participants with and without LV walked barefoot for four meters at a self-selected comfortable pace, starting upon a verbal cue from a quiet standing position and using the Tekscan High-Resolution Floor Mat System (Tekscan Inc., South Boston, MA, USA). After each trial, participants returned to a marked starting position. Three trials were performed under this condition, with guarded assistance provided as needed. Additionally, participants without LV underwent two other conditions: GI using a non-immersive low vision sight simulator (SS; Fork in the Road, Madison, WI, USA) and GI while immersed in Richie's Plank VR experience (see Figure 2B), specifically designed to evoke a fear of heights and falling. The VR condition was delivered using an HTC VIVE Cosmos Elite head-mounted display (HTC Corporation, Taiwan, China). The SS condition employed a non-immersive visual impairment simulator designed to reduce visual clarity and contrast, thereby mimicking low-vision conditions. The same gait initiation task instructions and verbal cues were used across all experimental conditions. Three trials were completed for each condition, with rest provided between trials as needed. All experimental procedures were completed within a single session lasting less than one hour.

https://doi.org/10.3390/healthcare14030400

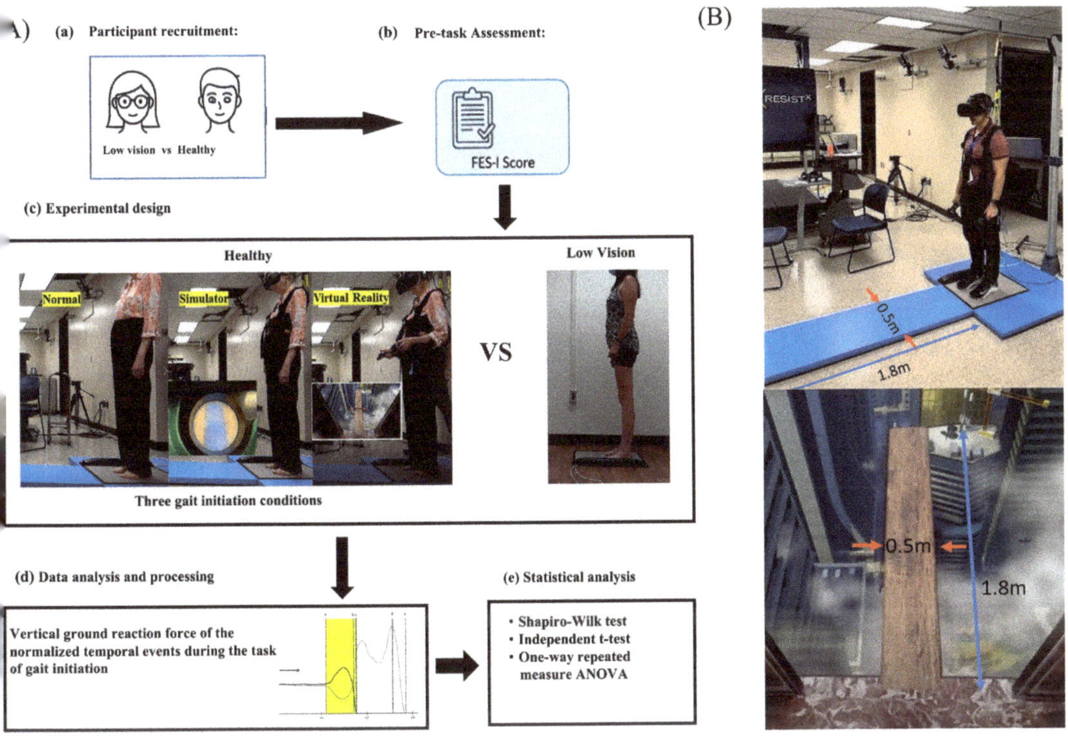

Figure 2. Proposed research pipeline and experimental setup. (**A**) The proposed research pipeline for evaluating the impact of visual and environmental constraints on gait initiation (GI). The framework includes: (**a**) Recruitment of healthy and low vision groups; (**b**) FOF assessment using the FES-I scale; (**c**) Experimental design comparing three GI conditions (normal, SS, and VR-induced height exposure) between groups; (**d**) Data acquisition of vertical ground reaction force using the Tekscan system; and (**e**) Statistical evaluation to verify data normality and compare group differences, illustrating the sequential research pipeline. (**B**) A healthy individual with HTC VIVE Cosmos Elite 3D VR system positioned on Tekscan High-Resolution Floor Mat for Richie's Plank experience.

2.3. Data Processing

Each temporal event of GI was captured by the vertical ground reaction force between swing and stance limbs with the Tekscan High-Resolution Floor Mat System. These temporal events of GI are illustrated in Figure 3.

To normalize temporal parameters of GI, the time from the onset of movement (Figure 3a) to stance limb toe-off (Figure 3e) was defined as 100% of the GI cycle (Figure 3). As such, relative temporal events are represented in percentages. The dependent variables are anticipation phase (AP), push-off phase (PO), anticipatory postural adjustment phase (APA), and double limb support time phase (DST) of both absolute and relative temporal events during GI. No kinematic data were collected in this study; all dependent variables were temporal events of gait initiation derived from vertical ground reaction forces.

https://doi.org/10.3390/healthcare14030400

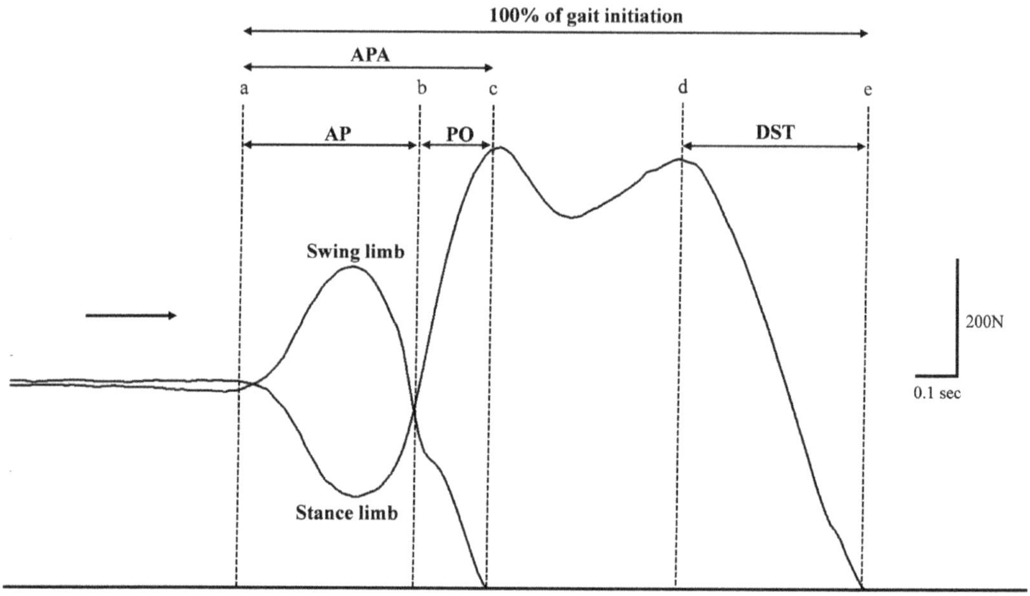

Figure 3. Vertical ground reaction force (Fz) of the temporal events during the task of gait initiation from one healthy individual (HK2). (a) Onset of movement, (b) Swing limb heel-off, (c) Swing limb toe-off, (d) Swing limb initial contact, and (e) Stance limb toe-off. The arrow indicates the direction of movement. Abbreviations: APA: anticipation postural adjustment phase; AP: anticipation phase; PO: push-off phase; DST: double limb support time phase.

2.4. Statistical Analysis

The Shapiro–Wilk test was conducted to identify the normality of all dependent variables, which include both absolute and relative temporal events as measured by vertical ground reaction forces during GI for both participants with and without LV. Additionally, Levene's test was employed to ensure the homogeneity of variance across groups, and this assumption was satisfied ($p > 0.05$).

An independent *t*-test was employed to assess whether there was a significant difference in the levels of concern about falling between participants with and those without LV. One-way repeated measure ANOVA was used to identify changes in SS and VR compared to a normal condition during the task of GI in participants without LV regarding AP, PO, APA, and DST of both absolute and relative temporal events. Post hoc analyses were conducted using the Bonferroni post hoc test. To compare participants with and without LV, we used an independent *t*-test to assess changes in AP, PO, APA, and DST for both absolute and relative temporal events. The significance level was set at $\alpha < 0.05$. All calculations were conducted using SPSS IBM version 28.

3. Results

3.1. Concerns About Falling in Individuals with LV

For the Falls Efficacy Scale International, the independent *t*-test showed that individuals with LV had significantly greater fear compared to healthy individuals (t (26) = −4.789, $p < 0.001$). Please refer to Figure 4.

https://doi.org/10.3390/healthcare14030400

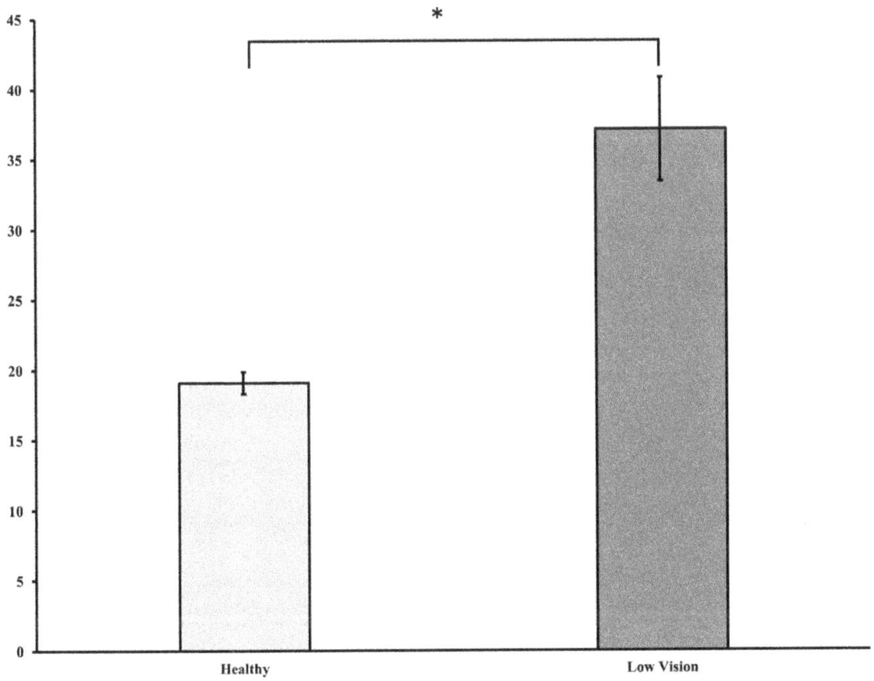

Figure 4. Falls Efficacy Scale International between healthy and low vision individuals. * $p < 0.05$.

3.2. Absolute Temporal Differences in VR, SS, and Normal Conditions Among Individuals Without LV

For APA, there was no significant multivariate main effect across the VR, SS, and normal conditions, $F(2, 12) = 2.222$, $p = 0.151$. However, a significant within-subject effect was observed (with sphericity assumed), $F(2, 26) = 4.271$, $p = 0.025$. The least significant difference test revealed that the VR condition resulted in a significantly prolonged APA time compared to the normal condition during GI ($p = 0.049$).

For AP, there was no significant multivariate main effect across the normal, SS, and VR conditions, $F(2, 12) = 1.784$, $p = 0.210$. For PO, a significant multivariate main effect was observed across the normal, SS, and VR conditions, $F(2, 12) = 8.424$, $p = 0.005$. However, no significant within-subject effects were detected (with sphericity assumed), $F(2, 26) = 1.650$, $p = 0.212$. The least significant difference test showed that the VR condition resulted in a significantly prolonged PO time compared to the normal condition during GI ($p = 0.033$). For the GI cycle, there was no significant multivariate main effect across the normal, SS, and VR conditions, $F(2, 12) = 1.627$, $p = 0.237$. Additionally, there were no significant within-subject effects (sphericity assumed), $F(2, 26) = 2.815$, $p = 0.078$. However, the least significant difference test revealed that the VR condition led to a significantly prolonged GI cycle compared to the normal condition during GI ($p = 0.049$).

For DST, data did not meet normality assumptions; therefore, this study employed a Friedman test. This test indicated significant differences across the normal, SS, and VR conditions during GI in individuals without LV, $\chi^2(2, N = 14) = 6.157$, $p = 0.046$. Subsequent post hoc analyses showed that the VR condition (mean = $0.511 \pm$ std = 0.718) had a significantly prolonged time compared to the SS condition (mean = $0.262 \pm$ std = 0.165) ($p = 0.018$).

https://doi.org/10.3390/healthcare14030400

3.3. Comparative Analysis of Absolute Temporal Events Between LV and Individuals Without LV

For APA, the independent *t*-test revealed that individuals with LV exhibited a significantly prolonged APA duration compared to both the normal ($p < 0.001$) and SS ($p < 0.001$) conditions. However, the APA duration in the LV group did not differ from the VR condition ($p = 0.320$). Please refer to Figure 5. The independent *t*-test also showed that individuals with LV had a significantly prolonged AP time compared to the normal ($p < 0.001$), SS ($p < 0.001$), and VR ($p = 0.049$) conditions. For PO, the independent *t*-test indicated no significant differences between individuals with LV and the normal ($p = 0.272$), SS ($p = 0.780$), or VR ($p = 0.601$) conditions. Regarding the GI cycle's duration, the independent *t*-test found that individuals with LV had a significantly prolonged duration compared to both the normal ($p < 0.001$) and SS ($p < 0.006$) conditions, but this duration was not different from the VR condition ($p = 0.830$). For DST, since the data did not meet the assumption of normality, a Mann–Whitney U test was used. The test revealed that individuals with LV did not significantly differ from individuals without LV in the normal ($U = 59.5$, $p = 0.077$), SS ($U = 59.5$, $p = 0.077$), or VR ($U = 100.5$, $p = 0.910$) conditions.

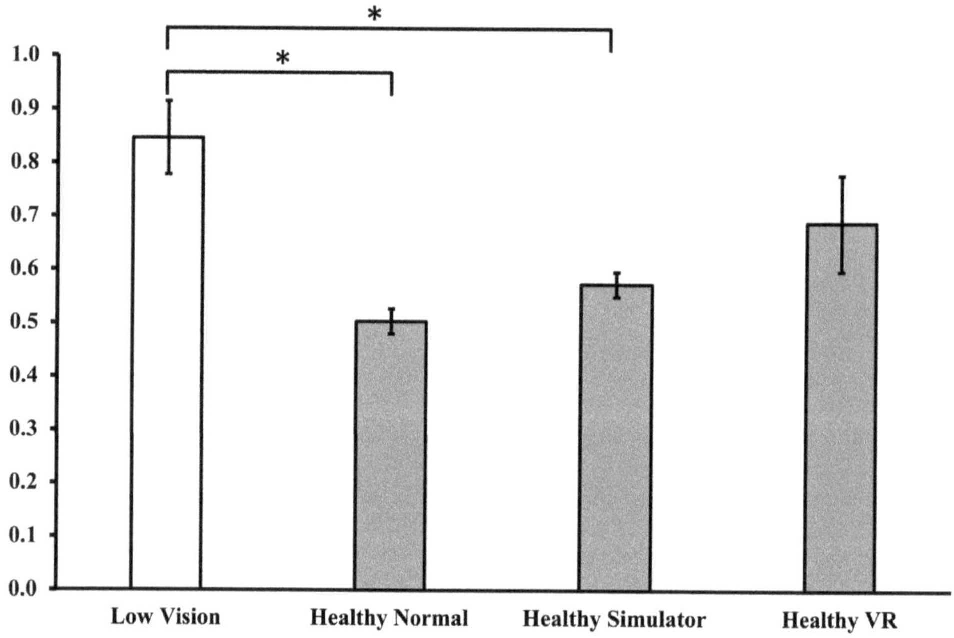

Figure 5. Anticipatory postural adjustment duration in absolute time between LV and healthy individuals. * $p < 0.05$. Abbreviations: VR (virtual reality).

3.4. Relative Temporal Differences in VR, SS, and Normal Conditions Among Individuals Without LV

For AP, there was no significant multivariate main effect across the normal, SS, and VR conditions, $F(2, 12) = 0.14$, $p = 0.986$. Similarly, no significant multivariate main effects were observed for PO and APA across the normal, SS, and VR conditions, with $F(2, 12) = 1.571$, $p = 0.248$, and $F(2, 12) = 0.234$, $p = 0.795$, respectively. For DST, since the data did not meet the assumption of normality, this study utilized a Friedman test. The test revealed no significant differences across the normal, SS, and VR conditions during GI in individuals without LV, $\chi^2(2, N = 14) = 3$, $p = 0.223$.

https://doi.org/10.3390/healthcare14030400

3.5. Comparative Analysis of Relative Temporal Events Between LV and Healthy Individuals

For APA, the independent *t*-test revealed that individuals with LV had a significantly prolonged APA duration compared to VR ($p = 0.004$), SS ($p < 0.001$), and normal ($p < 0.001$) conditions. Similarly, the independent *t*-test showed that individuals with LV had a significantly prolonged AP time when compared to the normal ($p < 0.001$), SS ($p < 0.001$), and VR ($p < 0.001$) conditions. However, for PO, the independent *t*-test indicated that there were no significant differences between individuals with LV and the VR ($p = 0.746$), SS ($p = 0.316$), and normal ($p = 0.399$) conditions.

For DST, as the data did not satisfy the assumption of normality, this study employed the Mann–Whitney U test. The results indicated that individuals with LV did not significantly differ from individuals without LV in the normal ($U = 127, p = 0.194$), SS ($U = 101$, $p = 0.910$), or VR ($U = 123, p = 0.265$) conditions.

4. Discussion

This study investigated the severity of fear-related changes in postural control in people with LV compared to age–gender-matched individuals without LV. The findings provide compelling evidence that individuals with LV demonstrate distinct postural control strategies that differ from individuals without LV and even from those individuals without LV in a fear-evoking VR environment. These unique strategies observed in individuals with LV reflect the unique challenges and the adaptations adopted by those with LV. This capacity of individuals with LV to adapt and adjust their postural control strategies in response to task and environmental demands has broader implications for fall prevention strategies and rehabilitation programs.

When assessing absolute temporal changes in the VR, SS, and normal conditions among individuals without LV, the AP remained unchanged, which is in contrast with the study's findings of significantly prolonged PO in the VR environment. The unchanged AP among participants without LV underlies the stability of postural control even during challenging conditions. However, the finding of prolonged PO emphasizes that even in the absence of visual impairments, fear-evoking stimuli such as fear of heights and falling can create hesitations and alterations in postural control strategies. This finding suggests that the significantly prolonged APA duration could be attributed to an increased duration of PO in response to a fear-evoking stimulus during the task of GI for individuals without LV. Additionally, the study's findings illustrated that the participants with LV demonstrated movement hesitations or adjustments comparable to participants without LV in the VR environment. Distinctly, however, participants with LV exhibit significantly longer AP duration compared to all conditions of participants without LV.

GI represents a critical transitional phase between quiet standing and dynamic walking, during which a stable postural equilibrium is intentionally disrupted. This transition is primarily governed by a feedforward motor program rather than reactive feedback-based control. As previously established, GI is mediated by APAs, characterized by reciprocal inhibition of the stance limb plantar flexors and activation of the dorsiflexors [33–36]. These coordinated muscle actions generate a posterior and lateral shift in the COP toward the swing limb, followed by a rapid forward transfer toward the stance limb to facilitate the transition from a static to a dynamic state (please see Figure 6). Because this process necessitates deliberate destabilization of balance, it may evoke fear and hesitation, particularly in individuals with low vision. Importantly, such hesitation is unlikely to reflect delayed sensory feedback processing; rather, it appears to manifest as a conservative modulation of the feedforward motor program. The present findings demonstrate a progressive reduction in stance limb unloading and swing limb loading under visually challenging conditions, indicating diminished weight shifting during APAs (please see Figure 7).

https://doi.org/10.3390/healthcare14030400

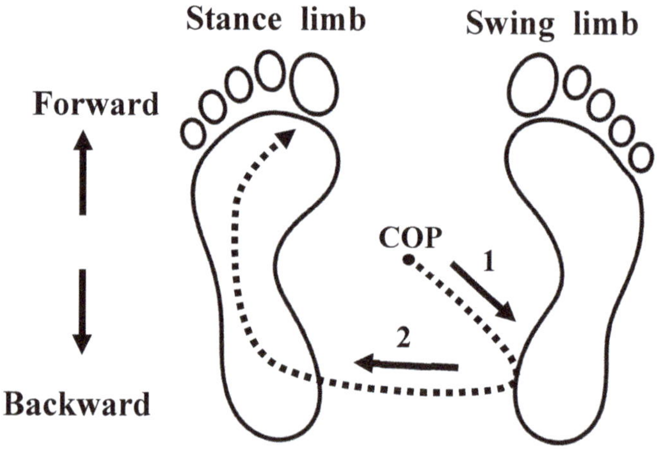

Figure 6. Dynamic weight shifting between the swing and stance limbs during gait initiation. 1. Backward center-of-pressure (COP) shift with weight transfer toward the swing limb (loading) and concurrent unloading of the stance limb. 2. Subsequent weight transfer toward the stance limb (loading) accompanied by unloading of the swing limb.

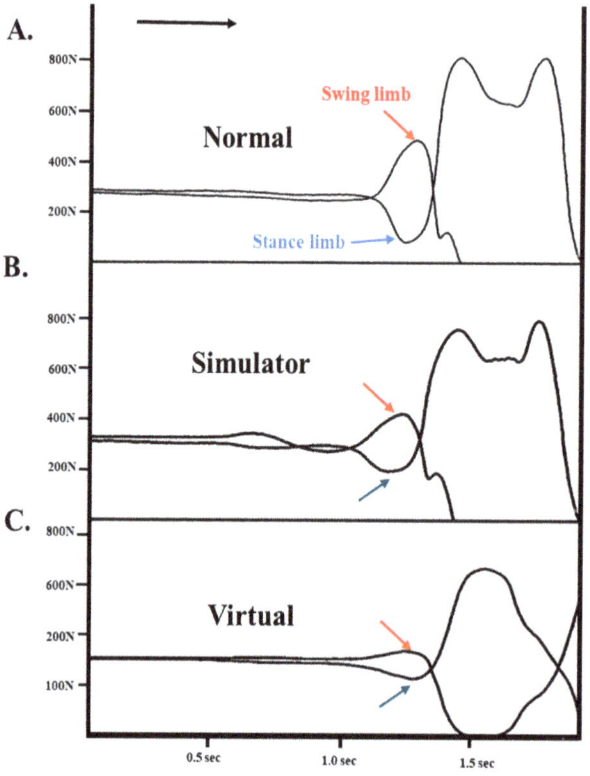

Figure 7. Vertical ground reaction forces of the stance and swing limbs during gait initiation under visually challenging conditions in healthy individuals. The figure illustrates a progressive reduction in stance limb unloading and swing limb loading during anticipatory postural adjustments across (**A**) normal, (**B**) SS, and (**C**) VR conditions.

https://doi.org/10.3390/healthcare14030400

Similar attenuations in COP excursion have been reported in populations with impaired balance control, such as frail older adults and individuals with hemiparesis, who adopt conservative anticipatory strategies to prioritize stability over mobility [33,36]. Notably, the movement strategies observed in individuals with low vision were comparable to those seen under fear-inducing virtual height conditions, characterized by constrained dynamic weight shifting. This quantitative reduction in anticipatory weight transfer likely reflects a chronic adaptive response to fear of falling, highlighting the severity and persistence of balance-related anxiety in the low-vision population.

These findings were reflected in the relative temporal events, in which people with LV exhibited a significantly prolonged APA duration, primarily due to an extended AP time compared to all conditions (VR, SS, and normal) observed in participants without LV. This finding further suggests that individuals with LV might experience even greater temporal hesitations than individuals without LV in fear-evoking virtual simulations during GI, suggesting that participants with LV exhibit greater FOF than those without LV. Concordantly, the participants in this study with LV reported greater concerns with falling on the FES-I compared to those without LV, agreeing with findings of previous studies assessing self-reported concerns with falling [32]. Interestingly, while participants without LV showed an extended PO in the VR condition, individuals with LV exhibited a longer AP duration, suggesting that individuals with LV employ distinct postural strategies to adapt to their fear before executing the first step from a static standing position (GI). However, most of the work previously has explored GI in other populations or has explored overall postural control, balance, or gait stability in individuals with LV, while limited work exists assessing the characteristics of GI in people with LV despite the known relationship of prolonged GI to multiple falls. GI has been strongly associated with vision and older adults demonstrate a delayed sensory reweighting process to compensate for VI [11]. Individuals diagnosed with VI demonstrate postural control mechanisms different from those of individuals without LV, which are further compensated by the remaining intact sensory systems [9,21,22,37–40]. If a delay in the sensory reweighting process exists in individuals with LV, individuals with LV may demonstrate prolonged APAs during GI.

Taken together, the present findings on GI in individuals with LV should be interpreted in light of the distinction between functional capacity and real-world performance. As these data were collected in a controlled laboratory environment, they primarily reflect participants' capacity under safe and predictable conditions. In daily community life, individuals with LV are exposed to additional contextual factors such as uneven surfaces, environmental obstacles, variable lighting, time constraints, and cognitive demands, which may further shape fear-related postural control strategies. Thus, while providing an important foundation for understanding the postural strategies during GI, these findings suggest the need for future research to examine how such strategies manifest in real-world settings. In addition, although kinematic data were not extracted in the present study, future investigations may incorporate kinematic analyses to further characterize movement strategies and fall-related mechanisms during APAs.

4.1. Clinical Implications

This present study's findings draw attention to the unique postural control strategies adopted by individuals with LV, suggesting the need for a tailored approach in low vision rehabilitation programs [41]. Prior research has shown that despite professional recommendations for preferred practice patterns proposed by the American Academy of Ophthalmology in 2017 [42], barriers to low vision rehabilitation hinder the utilization of low vision rehabilitation in regular ophthalmology practice [39]. Given the evident delays in APA during GI in these individuals, targeted interventions aiming to improve

https://doi.org/10.3390/healthcare14030400

postural control during a steady state walking and GI hold the potential to reduce the risks associated with FOF and falls.

Prior studies in LV interventions show the benefits of LV devices or aids, such as electronic magnifiers, electronic walking sticks, and smart glasses, which could act as compensatory strategies to address the functional needs of individuals with LV [43–45]. However, low vision rehabilitation needs to be multidisciplinary to address the multidimensional factors related to FOF in individuals with LV, especially since the provision of visual aids only for these individuals is ineffective in changing their FOF [46]. A recent systematic review in people with neurological disorders showed that a combination of gait training with lower limb training and balance exercises were effective in reducing FOF in individuals with Parkinson's disease, while individuals with multiple sclerosis also benefitted from the addition of home-based and leisure exercise in FOF reduction [47]. These principles extend naturally to stroke survivors, in whom FOF frequently exacerbates impaired GI. Inefficient APAs and inadequate limb loading not only hinder mechanical propulsion but also act as psychological barriers, reinforcing fear-related mobility restrictions. Consequently, stroke rehabilitation must evolve beyond static training to incorporate dynamic, task-specific interventions. By actively targeting APAs through controlled weight-shifting tasks and strategic GI protocols, clinicians may enhance the functional loading of the paretic limb [33]. Addressing these biomechanical foundations may therefore provide a dual benefit by improving physical stability while simultaneously reducing FOF that limits functional recovery. In addition to addressing the motor and physical aspects of FOF, the addition of cognitive behavioral therapy holds promise in reducing FOF and improving balance performance in older individuals with FOF [48]. These unique findings amongst different populations in which FOF is prevalent, however, underscore the need for more rigorous studies that explore specific low vision rehabilitation interventions that could positively influence FOF and subsequent fall risk in individuals with LV.

In addition to participating in physical exercise and strength training [42,49], more recent studies have explored the potential of training sensory reweighting and its potential role in addressing maladaptive postural control strategies in individuals with LV. Sensory reweighting programs may be integrated into standard low vision rehabilitation programs to help train the brain to more efficiently utilize intact sensory systems in the absence of adequate visual input. Specifically, given that the vestibular system is crucial for postural control, vestibular exercise programs may hold potential benefits for individuals with LV. After a 3-month vestibular stimulating exercise regime, the 28 individuals with visual impairments showed postural stability comparable to the 42 individuals without visual impairments in stabilometry tests with eyes closed [50]. LV rehabilitation emphasizes the importance of integrating sensory reweighting and vestibular exercise programs to enhance postural control, particularly as balance and vestibular exercises aim to improve the sensory reweighting process and may be beneficial for mitigating prolonged APAs in individuals with LV; however, further studies are needed to assess their effect on GI specifically.

4.2. Limitations

In addition to the small sample size, our study focused primarily on fear-evoking environments (fear of heights) in a controlled VR-simulated setting. Real-world scenarios pose different challenges and stimuli that were not replicated in this study. Future studies should explore the implications of these findings in larger samples and more varied and unpredictable settings to better understand the dynamic interaction of postural control, FOF, VI, and environment and task demands in individuals with LV. Although amplitude was not treated as a dependent variable in the present study, incorporating normalized amplitude

https://doi.org/10.3390/healthcare14030400

measures may help address inter-subject variability and enhance the comparability of gait-related outcomes across participants.

5. Conclusions

This study demonstrates that individuals with LV who self-report a FOF exhibit objectively impaired GI, characterized by significantly prolonged APAs. Our findings reveal that while fear-evoking environments cause temporary hesitations in sighted individuals, those with LV adopt a chronically conservative feedforward motor program, specifically lengthening the initial phase of postural preparation, referred to as the anticipation phase. Since vision plays a pivotal role in how we prepare and initiate movement, acting as one of the primary senses we use to safely navigate our environment, its impairment can markedly alter how individuals anticipate and interact with their physical environment during movement transitions that require deliberate destabilization of static balance, such as gait initiation. Consequently, these results suggest that proactive clinical referrals and multidisciplinary rehabilitation strategies incorporating sensory reweighting and vestibular training are essential to effectively address FOF, optimize postural control, and mitigate fall risks in individuals with LV.

Author Contributions: Conceptualization, M.K.; Methodology, M.K., P.K.G., G.B., T.C. and R.L.W.; Formal analysis, M.K., G.B., M.R.C., P.A. and T.C.; Investigation, M.K., P.K.G., G.B., M.R.C., P.A., T.C. and R.L.W.; Resources, M.K. and P.K.G.; Data curation, M.R.C. and P.A.; Writing—original draft, M.K.; Writing—review and editing, M.K., P.K.G., G.B., M.R.C., P.A., T.C. and R.L.W.; Visualization, M.K.; Supervision, M.K. and P.K.G.; Project administration, M.K. All authors have read and agreed to the published version of the manuscript.

Funding: This research received no external funding.

Institutional Review Board Statement: The study was conducted in accordance with the principles of the Declaration of Helsinki (1975, revised in 2013) and was reviewed and approved by the Institutional Review Board of the University of Texas Medical Branch (UTMB) prior to study initiation (approval code: IRB #21-0106, approved on 13 August 2021).

Informed Consent Statement: Written informed consent was obtained from all participants prior to participation in this study.

Data Availability Statement: The data presented in this study include de-identified human participant data derived from clinical electronic medical records (EPIC) and balance assessments. Due to ethical, legal, and privacy restrictions, the data are not publicly available. Data are available from the corresponding author upon reasonable request and subject to institutional and IRB regulations.

Conflicts of Interest: The authors declare no conflict of interest.

References

1. Rizzo, J.R.; Beheshti, M.; Hudson, T.E.; Mongkolwat, P.; Riewpaiboon, W.; Seiple, W.; Ogedegbe, O.G.; Vedanthan, R. The global crisis of visual impairment: An emerging global health priority requiring urgent action. *Disabil. Rehabil. Assist. Technol.* **2023**, *18*, 240–245. [CrossRef]
2. Rein, D.B.; Wittenborn, J.S.; Zhang, P.; Sublett, F.; Lamuda, P.A.; Lundeen, E.A.; Saaddine, J. The Economic Burden of Vision Loss and Blindness in the United States. *Ophthalmology* **2022**, *129*, 369–378. [CrossRef]
3. Nguyen, A.M.; Arora, K.S.; Swenor, B.K.; Friedman, D.S.; Ramulu, P.Y. Physical activity restriction in age-related eye disease: A cross-sectional study exploring fear of falling as a potential mediator. *BMC Geriatr.* **2015**, *15*, 64. [CrossRef]
4. Crews, J.E.; Chou, C.-F.; Stevens, J.A.; Saaddine, J.B. Falls Among Persons Aged ≥65 Years with and Without Severe Vision Impairment—United States, 2014. *Morb. Mortal. Wkly. Rep.* **2016**, *65*, 433–437. [CrossRef]
5. Reed-Jones, R.J.; Solis, G.R.; Lawson, K.A.; Loya, A.M.; Cude-Islas, D.; Berger, C.S. Vision and falls: A multidisciplinary review of the contributions of visual impairment to falls among older adults. *Maturitas* **2013**, *75*, 22–28. [CrossRef] [PubMed]

https://doi.org/10.3390/healthcare14030400

6. Ehrlich, J.R.; Hassan, S.E.; Stagg, B.C. Prevalence of Falls and Fall-Related Outcomes in Older Adults with Self-Reported Visi Impairment. *J. Am. Geriatr. Soc.* **2019**, *67*, 239–245. [CrossRef]
7. Young, W.R.; Williams, A.M. How fear of falling can increase fall-risk in older adults: Applying psychological theory to practi observations. *Gait Posture* **2015**, *41*, 7–12. [CrossRef] [PubMed]
8. Donoghue, O.A.; Ryan, H.; Duggan, E.; Finucane, C.; Savva, G.M.; Cronin, H.; Loughman, J.; Kenny, R.A. Relationship betwe fear of falling and mobility varies with visual function among older adults. *Geriatr. Gerontol. Int.* **2014**, *14*, 827–836. [CrossR [PubMed]
9. Yiou, E.; Caderby, T.; Delafontaine, A.; Fourcade, P.; Honeine, J.L. Balance control during gait initiation: State-of-the-art a research perspectives. *World J. Orthop.* **2017**, *8*, 815–828. [CrossRef]
10. Callisaya, M.L.; Blizzard, L.; Martin, K.; Srikanth, V.K. Gait initiation time is associated with the risk of multiple falls population-based study. *Gait Posture* **2016**, *49*, 19–24. [CrossRef]
11. Kimijanova, J.; Hirjakova, Z.; Bzduskova, D.; Hlavacka, F. Influence of vision on gait initiation and first step kinematics in you and older adults. *Physiol. Res.* **2021**, *70*, S409–S417. [CrossRef]
12. Sarlegna, F.R.; Sainburg, R.L. The roles of vision and proprioception in the planning of reaching movements. *Adv. Exp. Med. Bi* **2009**, *629*, 317–335. [CrossRef]
13. Ellmers, T.J.; Maslivec, A.; Young, W.R. Fear of Falling Alters Anticipatory Postural Control during Cued Gait Initiatio *Neuroscience* **2020**, *438*, 41–49. [CrossRef] [PubMed]
14. Errington, J.A.; Menant, J.C.; Suttle, C.M.; Bruce, J.; Asper, L.J. The effects of vertical yoked prisms on gait. *Investig. Ophthalm Vis. Sci.* **2013**, *54*, 3949–3956. [CrossRef] [PubMed]
15. Helbostad, J.L.; Vereijken, B.; Hesseberg, K.; Sletvold, O. Altered vision destabilizes gait in older persons. *Gait Posture* **200** *30*, 233–238. [CrossRef]
16. Raffegeau, T.E.; Young, W.R.; Fino, P.C.; Williams, A.M. A Perspective on Using Virtual Reality to Incorporate the Affectiv Context of Everyday Falls Into Fall Prevention. *JMIR Aging* **2023**, *6*, e36325. [CrossRef] [PubMed]
17. Suglia, V.; Brunetti, A.; Pasquini, G.; Caputo, M.; Marvulli, T.M.; Sibilano, E.; Della Bella, S.; Carrozza, P.; Beni, C.; Naso, D.; et a A Serious Game for the Assessment of Visuomotor Adaptation Capabilities during Locomotion Tasks Employing an Embodie Avatar in Virtual Reality. *Sensors* **2023**, *23*, 5017. [CrossRef]
18. Raffegeau, T.E.; Fawver, B.; Clark, M.; Engel, B.T.; Young, W.R.; Williams, A.M.; Lohse, K.R.; Fino, P.C. The feasibility of usin virtual reality to induce mobility-related anxiety during turning. *Gait Posture* **2020**, *77*, 6–13. [CrossRef]
19. Gomaa, Y.S.; Awad, M.I.; Emara, T.; Elbokl, A.; Al-Yahya, E.; ElMeligie, M.M. Role of virtual reality in examining the effect of fea of falling (FOF) on postural stability in individuals without and with Parkinson's disease in Egypt: A mixed-methods feasibilit study protocol. *BMJ Open* **2024**, *14*, e080592. [CrossRef]
20. Palazzo, L.; Suglia, V.; Grieco, S.; Buongiorno, D.; Brunetti, A.; Carnimeo, L.; Amitrano, F.; Coccia, A.; Pagano, G.; D'Addio, G et al. A Deep Learning-Based Framework Oriented to Pathological Gait Recognition with Inertial Sensors. *Sensors* **2025**, *25*, 26([CrossRef]
21. Friedrich, M.; Grein, H.J.; Wicher, C.; Schuetze, J.; Mueller, A.; Lauenroth, A.; Hottenrott, K.; Schwesig, R. Influence of pathologi and simulated visual dysfunctions on the postural system. *Exp. Brain Res.* **2008**, *186*, 305–314. [CrossRef]
22. Alghadir, A.H.; Alotaibi, A.Z.; Iqbal, Z.A. Postural stability in people with visual impairment. *Brain Behav.* **2019**, *9*, e01436 [CrossRef]
23. Cleworth, T.W.; Horslen, B.C.; Carpenter, M.G. Influence of real and virtual heights on standing balance. *Gait Posture* **2012** *36*, 172–176. [CrossRef]
24. Yardley, L.; Beyer, N.; Hauer, K.; Kempen, G.; Piot-Ziegler, C.; Todd, C. Development and initial validation of the Falls Efficacy Scale-International (FES-I). *Age Ageing* **2005**, *34*, 614–619. [CrossRef]
25. Dewan, N.; MacDermid, J.C. Fall Efficacy Scale-International (FES-I). *J. Physiother.* **2014**, *60*, 60. [CrossRef]
26. Hauer, K.; Yardley, L.; Beyer, N.; Kempen, G.; Dias, N.; Campbell, M.; Becker, C.; Todd, C. Validation of the Falls Efficacy Scale and Falls Efficacy Scale International in geriatric patients with and without cognitive impairment: Results of self-report and interview-based questionnaires. *Gerontology* **2010**, *56*, 190–199. [CrossRef]
27. Kuo, C.T.; Chen, D.R.; Chen, Y.M.; Chen, P.Y. Validation of the short falls efficacy scale-international for Taiwanese community-dwelling older adults: Associations with fall history, physical frailty, and quality of life. *Geriatr. Nurs.* **2021**, *42*, 1012–1018. [CrossRef] [PubMed]
28. Marques-Vieira, C.M.A.; de Sousa, L.M.M.; de Sousa, L.M.R.; Berenguer, S.M.A.C. Validation of the Falls Efficacy Scale—International in a sample of Portuguese elderly. *Rev. Bras. Enferm.* **2018**, *71*, 747–754. [CrossRef] [PubMed]
29. Yuki, K.; Asaoka, R.; Ono, T.; Awano-Tanabe, S.; Murata, H.; Tsubota, K. Evaluation of Fear of Falling in Patients with Primary Open-Angle Glaucoma and the Importance of Inferior Visual Field Damage. *Investig. Ophthalmol. Vis. Sci.* **2020**, *61*, 52. [CrossRef] [PubMed]

https://doi.org/10.3390/healthcare14030400

Chang, K.C.; Chen, H.S.; Horng, Y.S.; Liou, H.H.; Liang, H.W. Cross-cultural adaptation of the Taiwan Chinese version of the Falls Efficacy Scale-International for community-dwelling elderly individuals. *BMC Geriatr.* **2022**, *22*, 881. [CrossRef]
Palagyi, A.; Ng, J.Q.; Rogers, K.; Meuleners, L.; McCluskey, P.; White, A.; Morlet, N.; Keay, L. Fear of falling and physical function in older adults with cataract: Exploring the role of vision as a moderator. *Geriatr. Gerontol. Int.* **2017**, *17*, 1551–1558. [CrossRef]
da Silva, E.S.; Fischer, G.; da Rosa, R.G.; Schons, P.; Teixeira, L.B.T.; Hoogkamer, W.; Peyre-Tartaruga, L.A. Gait and functionality of individuals with visual impairment who participate in sports. *Gait Posture* **2018**, *62*, 355–358. [CrossRef] [PubMed]
Ko, M.; Bishop, M.D.; Behrman, A.L. Effects of limb loading on gait initiation in persons with moderate hemiparesis. *Top. Stroke Rehabil.* **2011**, *18*, 258–268. [CrossRef]
Brun, D.; Lafferty, M.J.; McKeon, A.; Goode, B.; Mulhausen, C.; Polk, P. Invariant characteristics of gait initiation. *Am. J. Phys. Med. Rehabil.* **1991**, *70*, 206–212. [CrossRef]
Brunt, D.; Liu, S.M.; Trimble, M.; Bauer, J.; Short, M. Principles underlying the organization of movement initiation from quiet stance. *Gait Posture* **1999**, *10*, 121–128. [CrossRef]
Ko, M.; Cole, M.; Vinyard, R. Age-related Control Strategies to Execute the First Step from Standing in Older Adults. *J. Clin. Mov. Sci. Hum.* **2018**, *22*, 1–5. [CrossRef]
Ray, C.T.; Horvat, M.; Croce, R.; Mason, R.C.; Wolf, S.L. The impact of vision loss on postural stability and balance strategies in individuals with profound vision loss. *Gait Posture* **2008**, *28*, 58–61. [CrossRef]
Tomomitsu, M.S.; Alonso, A.C.; Morimoto, E.; Bobbio, T.G.; Greve, J.M. Static and dynamic postural control in low-vision and normal-vision adults. *Clinics* **2013**, *68*, 517–521. [CrossRef] [PubMed]
Khimani, K.S.; Battle, C.R.; Malaya, L.; Zaidi, A.; Schmitz-Brown, M.; Tzeng, H.M.; Gupta, P.K. Barriers to Low-Vision Rehabilitation Services for Visually Impaired Patients in a Multidisciplinary Ophthalmology Outpatient Practice. *J. Ophthalmol.* **2021**, *2021*, 6122246. [CrossRef]
Parreira, R.B.; Grecco, L.A.C.; Oliveira, C.S. Postural control in blind individuals: A systematic review. *Gait Posture* **2017**, *57*, 161–167. [CrossRef] [PubMed]
Meyniel, C.; Bodaghi, B.; Robert, P.Y. Revisiting Vision Rehabilitation. *Front. Syst. Neurosci.* **2017**, *11*, 82. [CrossRef] [PubMed]
Fontenot, J.L.; Bona, M.D.; Kaleem, M.A.; McLaughlin, W.M., Jr.; Morse, A.R.; Schwartz, T.L.; Shepherd, J.D.; Jackson, M.L.; American Academy of Ophthalmology Preferred Practice Pattern Vision Rehabilitation Committee. Vision Rehabilitation Preferred Practice Pattern. *Ophthalmology* **2018**, *125*, P228–P278. [CrossRef] [PubMed]
Elsman, E.B.M.; van Rens, G.H.M.B.; van Nispen, R.M.A. Quality of life and participation of young adults with a visual impairment aged 18–25 years: Comparison with population norms. *Acta Ophthalmol.* **2019**, *97*, 165–172. [CrossRef]
Ehrlich, J.R.; Spaeth, G.L.; Carlozzi, N.E.; Lee, P.P. Patient-Centered Outcome Measures to Assess Functioning in Randomized Controlled Trials of Low-Vision Rehabilitation: A Review. *Patient-Patient-Centered Outcomes Res.* **2017**, *10*, 39–49. [CrossRef]
Markowitz, S.N. State-of-the-art: Low vision rehabilitation. *Can. J. Ophthalmol.* **2016**, *51*, 59–66. [CrossRef]
Haran, M.J.; Cameron, I.D.; Ivers, R.Q.; Simpson, J.M.; Lee, B.B.; Tanzer, M.; Porwal, M.; Kwan, M.M.S.; Severino, C.; Lord, S.R. Effect on falls of providing single lens distance vision glasses to multifocal glasses wearers: VISIBLE randomised controlled trial. *BMJ* **2010**, *340*, c2265. [CrossRef]
Abou, L.; Alluri, A.; Fliflet, A.; Du, Y.; Rice, L.A. Effectiveness of Physical Therapy Interventions in Reducing Fear of Falling Among Individuals with Neurologic Diseases: A Systematic Review and Meta-analysis. *Arch. Phys. Med. Rehabil.* **2021**, *102*, 132–154. [CrossRef]
8. Liu, T.-W.; Ng, G.Y.F.; Chung, R.C.K.; Ng, S.S.M. Cognitive behavioural therapy for fear of falling and balance among older people: A systematic review and meta-analysis. *Age Ageing* **2018**, *47*, 520–527. [CrossRef]
9. Elsman, E.B.M.; Al Baaj, M.; van Rens, G.H.M.B.; Sijbrandi, W.; van den Broek, E.G.C.; van der Aa, H.P.A.; Schakel, W.; Heymans, M.W.; de Vries, R.; Vervloed, M.P.J.; et al. Interventions to improve functioning, participation, and quality of life in children with visual impairment: A systematic review. *Surv. Ophthalmol.* **2019**, *64*, 512–557. [CrossRef]
0. Wiszomirska, I.; Kaczmarczyk, K.; Blazkiewicz, M.; Wit, A. The Impact of a Vestibular-Stimulating Exercise Regime on Postural Stability in People with Visual Impairment. *BioMed Res. Int.* **2015**, *2015*, 136969. [CrossRef] [PubMed]

https://doi.org/10.3390/healthcare14030400

healthcare

MDPI

Article

Perceptions of Fall Prevention and Engagement in Social Prescribing Activities Among Older Adults: A Cross-Sectional Study in Portugal

Cristiano Matos [1,2], Cristina Rosa Baixinho [2,3], Violeta Alarcão [1,4], Maria Adriana Henriques [1,2,5], Ricardo Oliveira Ferreira [1,2,5], Tiago Nascimento [1,2,5], Miguel Arriaga [1,6], Tatiana Alves [7,8,9], Paulo Nogueira [1,2,5] and Andreia Costa [1,2,5,*]

1 Instituto de Saúde Ambiental (ISAMB), Faculdade de Medicina, Universidade de Lisboa, 1600-190 Lisboa, Portugal; violeta_sabina_alarcao@iscte-iul.pt (V.A.); ahenriques@esel.pt (M.A.H.); rf@esel.pt (R.O.F.); tnascimento@esel.pt (T.N.); miguelarriaga@dgs.min-saude.pt (M.A.); pnogueira@medicina.ulisboa.pt (P.N.)
2 Nursing Research, Innovation and Development Centre of Lisbon (CIDNUR), Nursing School of Lisbon (Escola Superior de Enfermagem de Lisboa), University of Lisbon, 1600-190 Lisboa, Portugal; crbaixinho@esel.pt
3 Center for Innovative Care and Health Technology (ciTechcare), 2414-016 Leiria, Portugal
4 Centro de Investigação e Estudos de Sociologia (CIES-ISCTE), Instituto Universitário de Lisboa (ISCTE), 1649-026 Lisboa, Portugal
5 Laboratório Associado TERRA, Faculdade de Medicina, Universidade de Lisboa, 1649-028 Lisboa, Portugal
6 Católica Research Centre for Psychological—Family and Social Wellbeing (CRC-W), Faculdade de Ciências Humanas, Universidade Católica Portuguesa, 1649-023 Lisboa, Portugal
7 National Institute of Health Dr. Ricardo Jorge, Epidemiology Department, 1649-016 Lisboa, Portugal; tatiana.alves@insa.min-saude.pt
8 Instituto Politécnico de Setúbal, Escola Superior de Saúde, 2910-761 Setúbal, Portugal
9 Instituto de Ciências Sociais, Universidade de Lisboa, 1600-189 Lisboa, Portugal
* Correspondence: andreia.costa@esel.pt

Abstract

Background: Falls are a major cause of injury, functional decline, and reduced quality of life among older adults, posing a significant public health challenge. Social prescribing is gaining relevance in gerontology, offering structured strategies to engage individuals in preventive activities, including fall prevention strategies, through engagement in community-based activities. **Aim**: To examine older adults' perception of the relevance of personal protection and development activities (e.g., prevention against falling) and compare sociodemographic, behavioural, and engagement profiles between those who agree and those who disagree with its relevance. **Methods**: A cross-sectional study was conducted with 613 older adults aged 65–93 years. Data collection included sociodemographic, health-related, and behavioural/social engagement variables (including perceptions regarding the benefits of social prescribing and interest in community-based activities). For this analysis, participants were dichotomized based on their agreement with the relevance of personal protection and development activities (e.g., prevention against falling). Of the 569 participants included, 538 (94.5%) agreed with its relevance and 31 (5.5%) disagreed. Descriptive and exploratory analyses were conducted to compare the two groups across variables. Multivariate logistic regression analyses were conducted to explore independent predictors of agreement across sociodemographic, behavioural, social prescribing, and health-related variables. **Results**: Significant differences were observed between the groups in awareness of active ageing ($p = 0.018$), volunteering ($p < 0.001$), participation in social and community activities ($p < 0.001$), and hobbies like gardening, fishing, or cooking ($p = 0.002$). Those who agreed with the importance of personal protection and development activities were significantly more likely to value a range of initiatives, including social activities in recreational organizations, physical activity in the community (e.g., hiking), artistic and creative activities (e.g., visual arts, music), technical or technological activities (e.g., do-it-yourself, computers), and cultural enrichment activities (e.g., visiting museums), ($p < 0.001$). Multivariate analyses showed no effects of sociodemographic or health-related factors, whereas behavioural and engagement-related variables—including volunteering, hobbies, and several social prescribing activities—significantly predicted agreement with the relevance of personal protection and development activities. Discussion: The findings suggest that older adults who perceive fall prevention as relevant are more actively engaged in diverse health-promoting activities, including volunteering, hobbies, and community-based programmes. This pattern may reflect higher health literacy, stronger social networks, and proactive attitudes towards ageing. **Conclusions**: Perceptions of fall prevention are closely linked to broader patterns of engagement in health-promoting activities among older adults. Recognizing and addressing differences in how these activities are valued can inform more inclusive and targeted gerontological interventions.

Keywords: fall prevention; older adults; social prescribing; healthy ageing

1. Introduction

Falls are widely recognized as one of the most pressing public health problems affecting older adults [1], being a leading cause of injury and hospitalization, but also a determinant of disability, loss of independence, and premature mortality [1–4]. The consequences of falls extend far beyond the individual, with a substantial impact on families, caregivers, and healthcare systems, given the costs associated with emergency services, rehabilitation, and long-term care [5,6]. Furthermore, the psychological consequences, such as fear of falling and subsequent restriction of activities, contribute to functional decline, social isolation, and diminished quality of life [7].

The ageing of the population intensifies this challenge, with the proportion of older patients rising in recent decades [8,9]. Many of these individuals live with frailty, multimorbidity, or other age-related vulnerabilities, which increase the risk of falls [3,9]. Thus, fall prevention has emerged as a priority for promoting healthy ageing and ensuring the sustainability of health and social care systems [10,11], since it represents a considerable burden, generating high costs associated with emergency care, hospital admissions, rehabilitation, and long-term institutionalization, in addition to increasing demands on caregivers and community services [12,13].

The conventional fall prevention approaches have largely centred on clinical interventions, such as balance training, medication reviews, and home modifications, often applied after a first fall has occurred [14–16]. While effective to some extent, such approaches may overlook the broader determinants of falls, which include physical status but also psychosocial and environmental factors. Evidence increasingly supports the need for multidimensional interventions that go beyond the healthcare setting to embrace lifestyle, social participation, and community engagement as key protective factors [17,18].

In this context, social prescribing could be seen as an innovative model of care in primary health [19,20], which enables healthcare professionals to refer individuals to non-clinical services and community-based resources—including cultural, recreational, educational, and physical activities—aimed at addressing social determinants of health and enhancing well-being [20], promoting active engagement in different activities, and foster social connectedness, combat loneliness, and supports autonomy in later life [21,22]. These outcomes can be highly relevant for fall prevention, as stronger social networks, higher levels of physical activity, and improved Health Literacy (HL) have all been associated with reduced fall risk [23–25].

Recent studies have started to examine older adults' perceptions of social prescribing; Costa et al. (2024) conducted a national survey in Portugal showing high acceptance of social prescribing among older adults and identifying "personal protection and development" and "cultural enrichment" activities as particularly valued domains [19]. However, that study did not focus on fall prevention as a specific component within these activities, nor did it compare groups of older adults who agreed or disagreed with its relevance. In parallel, Percival et al. (2022) conducted a systematic review that concluded that, despite increasing recognition of social prescribing as a tool to enhance well-being in later life, there remains a lack of empirical studies exploring the mechanisms through which engagement in non-clinical activities translates into preventive outcomes [26].

Despite this, the integration of fall prevention strategies into social prescribing frameworks remains limited and insufficiently explored in research: little is known about how older adults themselves perceive the relevance of activities related to personal protection and development, such as fall prevention programmes, within the broader scope of community and social interventions.

The interplay between social capital, active ageing, and health literacy offers a valuable lens to interpret how older adults engage with preventive health initiatives. Social capital, through networks of trust, reciprocity, and social participation, creates the structural context in which individuals can access resources and support for healthy behaviours. Active ageing represents the functional outcome of this process, encompassing continued participation, autonomy, and self-fulfilment. Health literacy, in turn, acts as a mediating mechanism that enables older adults to interpret health information, make informed decisions, and translate social engagement into preventive action. Conceptually, these constructs are mutually reinforcing: higher health literacy fosters the capacity to mobilize social capital; social participation promotes active ageing; and engagement in active ageing behaviours further strengthens literacy and social connectedness.

The present study seeks to characterize the perceptions of older adults regarding the relevance of personal protection and development activities, with a particular focus on fall prevention. Specifically, it compares two groups—those who agree and those who disagree with the importance of such activities—across sociodemographic, health-related, and behavioural/social engagement variables (including social prescribing-related dimensions).

2. Materials and Methods

2.1. Study Design and Participants

The study employed a cross-sectional design with a representative sample of community-dwelling older adults in mainland Portugal. Data were collected between September and October 2022 through structured telephone interviews, conducted by trained interviewers using computer-assisted techniques. Participants were randomly selected from a pool of landline and mobile phone numbers generated by a specialized polling organization. The minimum required sample size was calculated using the OpenEpi tool (Version 3.01), assuming a 95% confidence level and a 5% margin of error. Considering a large population base of more than one million individuals and an assumed prevalence of 50%, which ensures maximum variability, the estimated minimum sample size was 384 participants. This calculation was supported by data from the most recent national census, indicating that approximately 2.3 million Portuguese residents are aged 65 years or older.

Eligibility criteria included being aged 65 years or older and living in mainland Portugal. Of those contacted, 613 individuals completed the survey, yielding a response rate of 74%. The structured questionnaire, developed by the research team based on prior studies and validated instruments on ageing and social prescribing [19], gathered information on sociodemographic (e.g., age, sex, marital status, education, employment situation), economic (e.g., perceived household financial situation), and health-related variables (e.g., presence of chronic conditions or disabilities, self-rated health).

The EQ-5D-3L instrument was used to assess health-related quality of life. It consists of a brief questionnaire and a visual analogue scale (VAS). The questionnaire includes five dimensions—mobility, self-care, usual activities, pain/discomfort, and anxiety/depression—each rated on a three-level scale (1 = no problems, 2 = some problems, 3 = extreme problems) [27]. It also assessed participants' perceptions of the benefits of social prescribing in terms of health and well-being, community cohesion, quality of care, and primary care functioning, and the usefulness of several categories of social prescribing activities (e.g., cultural, recreational, physical, artistic, technical, touristic, and personal protection/development activities), using a 7-point scale (1 = completely disagree to 7 = completely agree).

For this study, the variable "*usefulness of social prescribing activities related to personal protection and development activities (as prevention against falling)*" was used to dichotomize the sample into two groups: those who agreed with its relevance and those who disagreed. Individuals who selected a neutral response were excluded (n = 44), resulting in a final analytical sample of 569 older adults. Among these, 538 (94.5%) agreed with the relevance of personal protection and development activities, while 31 participants (5.5%) disagreed.

2.2. Ethical Considerations

All participants provided oral informed consent prior to participation. The study protocol was approved by the Ethics Committee of the Centro Académico de Medicina de Lisboa (Process no. 193/22) and adhered to the principles of the Declaration of Helsinki and the General Data Protection Regulation (GDPR).

2.3. Statistical Analysis

Data were analyzed using IBM SPSS Statistics 27.0 (IBM Corp., Armonk, NY, USA). Descriptive statistics, including frequencies, means, medians, standard deviations, and interquartile ranges, were used to characterize the sample. Group comparisons (agree vs. disagree) were conducted using Chi-square or Fisher's exact tests for categorical variables, depending on the distribution of cell frequencies. For continuous variables, data distributions were assessed through histograms, Q–Q plots, and the Shapiro–Wilk test. Variables meeting normality assumptions were compared using independent samples *t*-tests, while the Mann–Whitney U test was applied to non-normally distributed variables. Statistical significance was set at $p < 0.05$. Effect sizes were estimated using Cohen's d and eta squared (η^2). For analytical purposes, the Likert scale was treated as a continuous variable to allow calculation of descriptive statistics and group comparisons [28].

Although the unequal size of the agreement groups limited the stability of multivariate modelling, exploratory adjusted analyses were conducted using binary logistic regression to examine potential predictors of agreement with the relevance of personal protection and development activities.

3. Results

Sociodemographic characteristics of the sample are presented in Table 1. The majority of participants were aged between 65 and 74 years, married, and not working professionally. Educational levels were heterogeneous, with a predominance of basic and secondary education. Most respondents rated their household's financial situation as sufficient for their needs and their overall health as acceptable.

Table 1. Sociodemographic Characteristics.

Variable	Category	Agree (n = 538)	Disagree (n = 31)	*p*-Value
Sex	Male	281	15	Fisher's exact test: 0.715
	Female	257	0	
Age, years	65–74	355	23	Chi-square test 0.088
	75–84	163	5	
	>84	20	3	
Marital status	Married	349	17	Chi-square test: 0.347
	Other	189	14	
Educational level	No schooling or First cycle of basic education (4th grade)	148	6	Chi-square test 0.597
	Second or third cycle of basic education (6th–9th grade)	110	5	
	Secondary education (12th grade)	145	10	
	Bachelor's/Master's/PhD degree	135	10	
Employment situation	Working professionally	36	1	Fisher's exact test: 0.712
	Not working professionally	501	30	
Perceived household financial situation	Comfortable or very comfortable	150	9	Chi-square test 0.640
	Enough for needs	231	11	
	Difficult or very difficult	153	11	
Overall health rating	Good/Very good	168	10	Chi-square test 0.965
	Acceptable	273	15	
	Bad/Very bad	97	6	

When comparing the two groups—those who agreed versus those who disagreed with the relevance of personal protection and development activities—no statistically significant differences were found across sociodemographic variables, employment status, perceived financial situation, or self-rated health (all $p > 0.05$). This indicates that perceptions regarding the importance of fall prevention were not explained by basic demographic or economic characteristics.

Table 2 shows that most factors were perceived as contributing to active ageing, with consistently high mean scores across groups. Statistically significant differences were observed for volunteer activities ($p < 0.001$), social and community participation ($p < 0.001$), having hobbies ($p = 0.008$), and saving sufficient money for retirement ($p = 0.014$), which were rated higher contributor by the group that consider social prescribing activities of personal protection and development activities (as prevention against falling) as useful. No significant group differences were observed for health-related factors such as physical activity, diet, oral health, or mental health.

In Table 3, the perceived relevance of different social prescribing activities by group is represented. All activities were rated significantly higher by the group that considered social prescribing activities of personal protection and development activities as useful ($p < 0.001$ for all comparisons).

Table 2. Perceived Factors Contributing to Active Ageing.

ı Your Opinion, Which Factors Contribute to Ageing Actively?"	Mean (SD) Agree	Mean (SD) Disagree	Difference *p*-Value *t*-Test	Effect Size (Cohen's *d*)
ing free from chronic diseases such as diabetes or heart disease	3.08 (0.66)	3.23 (0.81)	0.143	
ing able to walk independently, even with physical limitations	3.15 (0.64)	3.26 (0.68)	0.343	
ıgaging in regular physical activity or exercise	3.26 (0.54)	3.26 (0.58)	0.960	
ting a healthy and balanced diet	3.33 (0.51)	3.16 (0.64)	0.179	
voiding the consumption of alcoholic beverages	3.00 (0.69)	2.90 (0.70)	0.505	
aintaining good oral health	3.32 (0.50)	3.19 (0.60)	0.303	
aving good mental health	3.42 (0.51)	3.26 (0.63)	0.185	
ot experiencing loneliness	3.29 (0.61)	3.13 (0.72)	0.233	
articipating in volunteer activities	3.22 (0.55)	2.84 (0.64)	<0.001	Medium 0.64
articipating in social and community activities	3.24 (0.52)	2.90 (0.54)	<0.001	Medium 0.64
aving hobbies such as gardening, fishing, or cooking	3.31 (0.54)	3.00 (0.68)	0.008	
ontinuing to learn new things	3.37 (0.51)	3.26 (0.51)	0.240	
aving sufficient money for retirement	3.22 (0.58)	2.90 (0.70)	0.014	
Iaving adequate housing	3.35 (0.51)	3.13 (0.72)	0.113	

Responses were collected on a 7-point Likert scale. For analytical purposes, the Likert scale was treated as a continuous variable to allow calculation of means and group comparisons.

Table 3. Relevance of different social prescribing activities by group—differences and correlation.

Relevance of Different Social Prescribing Activities by Group	Median—IQR Agree	Median—IQR Disagree	Difference *p*-Value Mann–Whitney	Effect Size (eta Square)
Cultural enrichment (e.g., visiting museums)	6.16 (0.91)	3.97 (2.12)	<0.001	Small $\eta^2 = 0.017$
Recreational/social activities	5.63 (1.34)	2.97 (1.64)	<0.001	Small $\eta^2 = 0.018$
Physical activity in community (e.g., hiking)	5.90 (1.22)	3.65 (2.09)	<0.001	Small $\eta^2 = 0.014$
Artistic/creative activities (e.g., music, visual arts)	5.65 (1.36)	3.23 (1.73)	<0.001	Small $\eta^2 = 0.016$
Technical/technological activities (e.g., DIY, computers)	5.80 (1.30)	3.29 (1.67)	<0.001	Small $\eta^2 = 0.019$
Touristic activities (e.g., excursions)	5.71 (1.37)	2.77 (1.67)	<0.001	Small $\eta^2 = 0.019$

Responses were collected on a 7-point Likert scale. For analytical purposes, the Likert scale was treated as a continuous variable to allow calculation of means and group comparisons.

Quality of life scores assessed by the EQ-5D-3L instrument for both groups are shown in Table 4. Perceived health state expressed with Index and VAS were very similar between groups, with no significant differences ($p = 0.981$ and $p = 0.659$).

Across the five EQ-5D dimensions—mobility, self-care, usual activities, pain/discomfort, and anxiety/depression—both groups presented comparable distributions. The majority of participants reported no problems with mobility, self-care, and usual activities, although a considerable proportion indicated some difficulties with pain/discomfort and anxiety/depression. No statistically significant differences emerged between groups in any of these dimensions (all $p > 0.05$).

Table 4. Quality Life Scores.

Dimension		Agree (n = 538)	Disagree (n = 31)	*p*-Value
Perceived health state (index) Mean (SD)		0.83 (0.20)	0.82 (0.18)	*t*-test $p = 0.981$
Perceived health status (VAS) Mean (SD)		70.65 (23.48)	72.54 (20.98)	*t*-test $p = 0.659$
Mobility	No problems	339 (63.01%)	23 (74.19%)	Fisher exact $p = 0.252$
	Some/Extreme problems	199 (36.98%)	8 (25.81%)	
Self-care	No problems	502 (93.31%)	29 (93.55%)	Fisher exact $p = 1.000$
	Some/Extreme problems	36 (6.68%)	2 (6.45%)	
Usual activities	No problems	420 (78.07%)	24 (77.42%)	Chi-square $p = 1.000$
	Some/Extreme problems	118 (21.93%)	7 (22.58%)	
Pain/discomfort	No problems	239 (44.43%)	12 (38.71%)	Chi-square $p = 0.581$
	Some/Extreme problems	299 (55.58%)	19 (61.29%)	
Anxiety/depression	No problems	363 (67.47%)	18 (58.06%)	Chi-square $p = 0.427$
	Some/Extreme problems	175 (32.52%)	12 (41.94%)	

The logistic regression assessing whether sociodemographic characteristics predicted agreement with the relevance of personal protection and development activities (including fall prevention) showed that none of the variables were significant predictors of the outcome: sex ($p = 0.677$), age ($p = 0.575$), marital status ($p = 0.875$), educational level ($p = 0.195$), employment status ($p = 0.827$), perceived financial situation ($p = 0.627$), and self-rated health ($p = 0.842$). The logistic regression model did not improve upon the null model, suggesting that sociodemographic factors do not account for the differences in perceptions observed. This is consistent with the univariate findings and supports the interpretation that attitudes toward fall prevention are not shaped by basic demographic or economic characteristics.

Regarding perceived factors contributing to active ageing, the logistic regression revealed three contributors to active ageing that independently predicted agreement with the relevance of personal protection and development activities. Perceiving volunteering as important was the strongest predictor (OR = 4.15, $p < 0.001$), followed by having hobbies such as gardening, fishing, or cooking (OR = 2.46, $p = 0.015$). Regular physical activity showed a modest negative association (OR = 0.31, $p = 0.006$). All other perceived contributors to active ageing were non-significant and did not enter the model. The final logistic regression model explained approximately 12.1% according to the Nagelkerke R^2, indicating a small explanatory capacity for the predictors included. The logistic regression model explained approximately 12.1% according to the Nagelkerke R^2, indicating a small explanatory capacity for the predictors included.

In the perceived relevance of different social prescribing activities, the logistic regression identified four activity domains that predicted agreement with the relevance of personal protection and development activities. Social activities in recreational associations emerged as a significant predictor (OR = 1.62, $p < 0.001$), indicating that individuals who value social participation are more likely to recognize the importance of fall-prevention-related initiatives. Technical or technological activities, such as do-it-yourself or computer use also showed a positive association (OR = 1.35, $p = 0.031$), suggesting that engagement in practical or skill-building tasks aligns with valuing preventive approaches. Cultural enrichment activities, including museum or monument visits, demonstrated a smaller but noteworthy effect (OR = 1.28, $p = 0.080$), while touristic activities such as excursions remained a strong and consistent predictor across steps (OR = 1.67, $p = 0.001$). All other activity domains were not retained in the final model. The final logistic regression model explained approximately 52.2% according to the Nagelkerke R^2, indicating a moderate to strong explanatory capacity for the predictors included.

Regarding quality-of-life variables assessed through the EQ-5D-3L, the logistic regression analysis showed that none of the dimensions—mobility, self-care, usual activities, pain/discomfort, or anxiety/depression—significantly predicted agreement with the relevance of personal protection and development activities (all $p > 0.20$). In addition, neither perceived health state (EQ-5D index score) nor self-rated health status (EQ-5D VAS score) showed any meaningful association with the outcome, indicating that older adults' agreement levels were not influenced by their general health perception or subjective health evaluation. Overall, these findings suggest that perceptions of the importance of personal protection and fall-prevention activities are not shaped by self-reported health status, functional ability, or perceived health quality, but instead appear to be driven by behavioural and engagement-related factors.

4. Discussion

The older adults' perceptions of the relevance of personal protection and development activities, such as fall prevention, were examined and compared between individuals who agreed with their importance to those who did not. Significant differences were observed across behavioural and social engagement variables, including awareness of active ageing, volunteering, participation in social and community activities, and involvement in hobbies such as gardening, fishing, or cooking. Moreover, older adults who valued fall prevention were more likely to recognize the usefulness of a wide range of social prescribing initiatives, including recreational, physical, artistic, technological, and cultural activities.

These results suggest that perceptions of fall prevention are closely intertwined with broader health-promoting behaviours and attitudes. Older adults who acknowledge the importance of preventing falls appear to adopt a more proactive approach to ageing, reflected in their greater social participation and community engagement. This pattern is consistent with evidence linking health literacy and positive attitudes toward ageing with increased adherence to preventive behaviours and improved health outcomes [24]. Participants who agreed with the importance of fall prevention rated certain active ageing factors—such as volunteering, social participation, and hobbies—more positively than those who did not consider fall prevention relevant. This consistent pattern suggests that perceiving fall prevention as important may reflect a broader understanding of "active ageing," encompassing autonomy, engagement, and personal fulfilment. For these individuals, preventive strategies appear to be viewed not as restrictive or risk-focused, but rather as enabling continued participation, independence, and well-being in later life. These findings underscore the importance of framing prevention as a component of active and healthy ageing, rather than solely as a response to vulnerability or risk.

Beyond conceptual alignment, several psychosocial and cultural factors may explain why some older adults place less emphasis on fall prevention. Previous studies have shown that acknowledging the risk of falling can be perceived as an admission of frailty, dependence, or ageing itself—conditions often stigmatized in many cultures [29,30]. As a result, some individuals may distance themselves from preventive messages to preserve a sense of autonomy and invulnerability. This response aligns with the notion of "positive denial," whereby older adults prefer to identify as active and self-reliant rather than at risk. Moreover, cultural norms that emphasize independence and productivity in later life may further discourage engagement in interventions framed explicitly around vulnerability or risk reduction.

A similar pattern was observed in the assessment of social prescribing activities (Table 3), where those who considered fall prevention relevant also attributed greater usefulness to all other types of community-based activities. This consistent association suggests that older adults who value fall prevention tend to recognize broader benefits in participating in social, cultural, and recreational initiatives. For these individuals, engagement in such activities may represent both an enjoyable and purposeful means of maintaining autonomy, social connection, and overall well-being. This pattern highlights that preventive and health-promoting motivations are not mutually exclusive but rather intertwined within a holistic understanding of active ageing. Consequently, communication strategies should frame fall-prevention initiatives as empowering, enriching, and socially meaningful experiences that support independence and participation, rather than as narrowly corrective or risk-avoidance measures.

The association between valuing fall prevention and involvement in volunteering and community-based activities highlights the role that social capital can have in shaping health behaviours [31]. Some studies have emphasized the importance of education and social engagement in fall prevention, highlighting that preventive education for older adults and their caregivers is critical and that social participation enhances the effectiveness of interventions. Educational strategies increase awareness of risk factors, improve self-management skills, and foster confidence in adopting preventive behaviours, while social engagement provides motivation, peer support, and opportunities to integrate these behaviours into daily life. Evidence suggests that when educational initiatives are combined with community participation, they not only improve knowledge but also translate into greater adherence to preventive practices and sustained reductions in fall risk [32,33]. Social prescribing aims to strengthen these networks by facilitating access to meaningful activities that promote autonomy, reduce isolation, and support functional capacity in later life [26,34]. Our findings suggest that individuals who already recognize the importance of fall prevention may be more receptive to such interventions, while those who dismiss their relevance could represent a harder-to-reach subgroup at greater risk.

From a theoretical perspective, according to the Transtheoretical Model, individuals who do not recognize the relevance of fall prevention may be in the precontemplation stage, characterized by low awareness of personal risk and limited readiness to adopt preventive behaviours [35]. Similarly, within the framework of the Health Belief Model (Rosenstock, 1974), these individuals may perceive low susceptibility to falls or low perceived benefits of preventive action, which in turn reduces their motivation to engage in fall-prevention initiatives [36]. Understanding this stage of readiness and perception of risk can help tailor interventions, for instance, by emphasizing positive outcomes such as autonomy and confidence rather than focusing exclusively on risk reduction.

Tailored strategies are therefore needed to engage this population, for example, through targeted communication campaigns, peer-led initiatives, or low-threshold community programmes. Community-based programmes, such as the STEADI initiative, illustrate the potential of combining multifactorial risk assessments with educational and community resources, showing effectiveness in reducing fall-related hospitalizations [37]. This type of collaboration resonates with the principles of social prescribing and reinforces its applicability in fall prevention [37]. Although no significant differences were found between groups regarding mobility levels, the descriptive patterns suggest that individuals with lower mobility may nonetheless express openness to cultural, recreational, and even physical activities within the community [38], indicating a willingness to maintain autonomy and social participation, provided that activities are adapted to functional capacity and accessible in their format. Future studies should examine in greater depth how mobility limitations interact with perceptions of social prescribing and identify the types of activities most valued by those with restricted physical function.

The multivariate findings reinforce that perceptions of the relevance of personal protection and development activities are not shaped by sociodemographic or health-related factors, but rather by behavioural and engagement-related characteristics. Older adults who value volunteering, hobbies, and a range of social prescribing activities were significantly more likely to recognize the importance of these preventive initiatives, suggesting that proactive engagement in community and leisure activities reflects a broader orientation toward active and autonomous ageing. In contrast, self-rated health, functional limitations and demographic attributes showed no meaningful influence, indicating that attitudes toward fall prevention arise less from objective health status and more from lifestyle patterns, interests, and existing social connectedness. This highlights the importance of integrating fall-prevention messages within socially meaningful and engaging contexts rather than relying solely on traditional risk-based communication.

The results also highlight the multidimensional nature of falls, which emphasizes that prevention must go beyond risk factors to encompass physical, social, and environmental determinants [8,39]. Participants who valued fall prevention also expressed greater interest in cultural, creative, and technological activities, suggesting that preventive behaviours are embedded in a wider lifestyle that promotes cognitive stimulation, social connectedness, and active ageing. However, participation in preventive programmes is often limited by individual barriers, such as denial or fear of being a burden, as well as community-level constraints, including transportation difficulties and limited resources [40]. Recognizing and addressing these obstacles is essential, since overcoming them directly supports the World Health Organization's definition of healthy ageing, which places functional ability and active participation in society at the core of ageing policies [41]. Future studies should associate falls and fear of falling with activities performed associated with social prescription.

Another key implication concerns health literacy: the differences observed between groups may reflect varying levels of knowledge, awareness, and confidence in managing health risks. Low health literacy has been linked to reduced engagement in preventive care, poorer self-management, and higher vulnerability to adverse outcomes, including falls [24,42]. A review that aimed to explore and synthesize the current evidence regarding the role of HL in enhancing fall prevention in hospital and community settings concludes that HL can be increased through tailored information, verbal debriefing, interactive communication, and culturally adapted interventions. Low HL impedes the understanding of education, engaging interventions, and using technological devices in implementing fall-prevention interventions [24]. Therefore, interventions to promote fall prevention within social prescribing should not only provide access to activities but also address underlying literacy gaps, empowering older adults to recognize the value of preventive behaviours. Thus, combining fall-prevention education with accessible community-based opportunities may represent a dual pathway to strengthen health literacy and social capital simultaneously.

The results suggest that social prescribing should be integrated into nursing care as a person-centred strategy to promote physical activity, prevent social isolation, and address key risk factors for falls. This approach also supports health literacy and facilitates referrals to appropriate community resources. By incorporating social prescribing into their practice, nurses can broaden fall-prevention interventions, enhance patient engagement, strengthen local support networks, and ultimately contribute to the preservation of autonomy and quality of life.

Finally, the findings have implications for health and social policy. In contexts where healthcare systems remain focused on secondary care, integrating fall prevention into primary care and community-based services is critical [43,44]. Social prescribing can serve as a bridge between health and social sectors, offering scalable and sustainable strategies to mitigate fall risk and support functional independence. Ensuring equitable access and tailoring interventions to those less convinced of their relevance will be essential to maximize impact.

Limitations

This study has some limitations. First, because this study used a cross-sectional design, it can only identify associations and not establish causal relationships between perceptions of fall prevention and engagement in health-promoting activities. It is therefore not possible to determine whether valuing fall prevention leads to greater participation in such activities, whether participation fosters greater awareness of fall prevention, or whether both are influenced by other underlying factors. Second, the small size of the "disagree" group limits statistical power for some analyses and may reduce the generalizability of subgroup comparisons. The authors acknowledge that future studies with larger samples could benefit from a multivariate logistic regression model to further assess independent predictors of agreement on the usefulness of fall prevention. In addition, self-reported data are subject to recall and social desirability biases. The study did not include objective data on participants' fall history or clinical risk of falling, which limits the ability to contextualize perceptions of fall prevention in relation to actual experiences or needs. Future studies should explore longitudinal associations between perceptions of fall prevention and actual participation in social prescribing activities, as well as evaluate interventions designed to shift perceptions among those less convinced of their relevance. Additionally, qualitative research could provide richer insights into the reasons why some older adults undervalue fall prevention, helping to design tailored and culturally sensitive approaches. A key strength of this study lies in its large and diverse sample of older adults, which allowed for meaningful comparisons across sociodemographic and behavioural variables. The inclusion of a wide range of activity types also provides a nuanced understanding of how perceptions of fall prevention relate to broader patterns of engagement in health-promoting behaviours.

5. Conclusions

This study highlights that older adults who recognize the importance of personal protection and development activities, such as fall prevention, are more actively engaged in a wide range of health-promoting initiatives, including volunteering, hobbies, and community-based programmes. These findings suggest that perceptions of fall prevention are not isolated but integrated into broader patterns of proactive ageing, supported by higher health literacy and stronger social networks.

To maximize the potential of social prescribing in gerontology, it is crucial to raise awareness about the value of preventive activities among those less inclined to recognize their relevance. Multifactorial interventions, exercise programmes, and community engagement are all critical components of fall prevention that can be facilitated through social prescribing. Tailored strategies that enhance health literacy, expand access to community resources, and foster inclusive participation may contribute to reducing fall risk, improving quality of life, and supporting healthy ageing at a population level. Further research is needed to explicitly evaluate the impact of social prescribing on fall prevention outcomes among older adults.

The findings suggest that communication about fall prevention should be reframed to emphasize autonomy, confidence, and continued participation rather than vulnerability or risk. Health professionals—particularly nurses and primary care teams—can integrate motivational approaches and person-centred dialogue to align preventive messages with older adults' values and self-perceptions. Community programmes may also benefit from embedding fall-prevention activities within broader social prescribing initiatives, such as cultural or recreational events, to reduce stigma and increase engagement. Tailoring materials to different levels of health literacy, using peer-led communication, and presenting prevention as a way to "stay active and independent" rather than "avoid falling" may further enhance participation and adherence.

Author Contributions: Conceptualization, A.C., M.A.H. and M.A.; Methodology, A.C., C.M., P.N., T.A. and C.R.B.; Software, C.M.; Validation, V.A. and C.R.B. Formal analysis, C.M. and P.N.; Investigation, M.A.H.; Resources, T.N. and V.A.; Data curation, C.M.; Writing—original draft preparation C.M.; Writing—review and editing, A.C., M.A.H., V.A., T.N., M.A., C.R.B., T.A., R.O.F. and P.N.; Supervision, A.C. and R.O.F.; Project administration, A.C. and P.N.; Funding acquisition, AC. All authors have read and agreed to the published version of the manuscript.

Funding: This study is part of the research programme of the General Foundation of the University of Salamanca, through the International Centre on Aging (CENIE), within the framework of the Programme for a Longevity Society (0551_PSL_6_E), a project co-financed by the European Regional Development Fund (ERDF) through the Interreg VA Spain-Portugal Programme (POCTEP) 2014–2020.

Institutional Review Board Statement: This study was approved by the Ethics Committee of the Centro Académico de Medicina de Lisboa (Process number 193/22) 15 September 2022 and complied with the ethical principles in the Declaration of Helsinki, and the General Data Protection Regulation (GDPR).

Informed Consent Statement: Informed consent was obtained from all subjects involved in the study.

Data Availability Statement: The data presented in this study are available on reasonable request from the corresponding author due to confidentiality and privacy restrictions. In accordance with the informed consent provided to participants, the responses are stored securely, accessible only to the research team, and will be deleted five years after publication of the articles resulting from the study, in compliance with applicable data protection legislation.

Conflicts of Interest: The authors declare no conflicts of interest.

eferences

Vaishya, R.; Vaish, A. Falls in older adults are serious. *Indian J. Orthop.* **2020**, *54*, 69–74. [CrossRef] [PubMed]

Malmivaara, A.; Heliövaara, M.; Knekt, P.; Reunanen, A.; Aromaa, A. Risk factors for injurious falls leading to hospitalization or death in a cohort of 19,500 adults. *Am. J. Epidemiol.* **1993**, *138*, 384–394. [CrossRef]

Pitchai, P.; Dedhia, H.B.; Bhandari, N.; Krishnan, D.; D'Souza, N.R.J.; Bellara, J.M. Prevalence, risk factors, circumstances for falls and level of functional independence among geriatric population-A descriptive study. *Indian J. Public Health* **2019**, *63*, 21–26. [CrossRef] [PubMed]

Toyabe, S. World Health Organization fracture risk assessment tool in the assessment of fractures after falls in hospital. *BMC Health Serv. Res.* **2010**, *10*, 106. [CrossRef] [PubMed]

Tzeng, H.-M.; Yin, C.-Y. Inpatient falls: The impact of family and personal caregivers. *Appl. Nurs. Res.* **2009**, *22*, 159–165. [CrossRef]

Faes, M.C.; Reelick, M.F.; Joosten-Weyn Banningh, L.W.; Gier Mde Esselink, R.A.; Olde Rikkert, M.G. Qualitative study on the impact of falling in frail older persons and family caregivers: Foundations for an intervention to prevent falls. *Aging Ment. Health* **2010**, *14*, 834–842. [CrossRef]

Jørstad, E.C.; Hauer, K.; Becker, C.; Lamb, S.E.; Group, P. Measuring the psychological outcomes of falling: A systematic review. *J. Am. Geriatr. Soc.* **2005**, *53*, 501–510. [CrossRef]

World Health Organization. *Falls [Internet]*; World Health Organization: Geneva, Switzerland, 2021. Available online: https://www.who.int/news-room/fact-sheets/detail/falls (accessed on 13 October 2025).

Peel, N.M. Epidemiology of falls in older age. *Can. J. Aging/La Rev. Can. Du Vieil.* **2011**, *30*, 7–19. [CrossRef]

10. Ungar, A.; Rafanelli, M.; Iacomelli, I.; Brunetti, M.A.; Ceccofiglio, A.; Tesi, F.; Marchionni, N. Fall prevention in the elderly. *Clin. Cases Miner. Bone Metab.* **2013**, *10*, 91.

11. Pfortmueller, C.A.; Lindner, G.; Exadaktylos, A.K. Reducing fall risk in the elderly: Risk factors and fall prevention, a systematic review. *Minerva Med.* **2014**, *105*, 275–281.

12. James, S.L.; Lucchesi, L.R.; Bisignano, C.; Castle, C.D.; Dingels, Z.V.; Fox, J.T.; Hamilton, E.B.; Henry, N.J.; Krohn, K.J.; Liu, Z.; et The global burden of falls: Global, regional and national estimates of morbidity and mortality from the Global Burden of Dise Study 2017. *Inj. Prev.* **2020**, *26* (Suppl. S2), i3–i11. [CrossRef] [PubMed]
13. Cotter, P.E.; Timmons, S.; O'Connor, M.; Twomey, C.; O'Mahony, D. The financial implications of falls in older people for an ac hospital. *Ir. J. Med. Sci.* **2006**, *175*, 11–13. [CrossRef] [PubMed]
14. Noohu, M.M.; Dey, A.B.; Hussain, M.E. Relevance of balance measurement tools and balance training for fall prevention in ol adults. *J. Clin. Gerontol. Geriatr.* **2014**, *5*, 31–35. [CrossRef]
15. Suen, J.; Narayan, S.; Seppala, L.J.; van der Velde, N.; Sherrington, C.; Sutcliffe, K.; Cameron, I.D.; Kneale, D.; Dyer, S. Features of successful medication review and deprescribing interventions for fall prevention in residential aged care facilities: intervention component analysis of an updated systematic review. *Age Ageing* **2025**, *54*, afaf230. [CrossRef]
16. Cumming, R.G.; Thomas, M.; Szonyi, G.; Frampton, G.; Salkeld, G.; Clemson, L. Adherence to occupational therapist recomme dations for home modifications for falls prevention. *Am. J. Occup. Ther.* **2001**, *55*, 641–648. [CrossRef]
17. MacCulloch, P.A.; Gardner, T.; Bonner, A. Comprehensive fall prevention programs across settings: A review of the literatu *Geriatr. Nurs.* **2007**, *28*, 306–311. [CrossRef]
18. Fordham, B.; Williamson, E. The Role of Social Prescribers in Engaging Older Adults in Strength and Balance Training After Bei Discharged From Physiotherapy Rehabilitation: A Qualitative Investigation. *Health Soc. Care Community* **2025**, *2025*, 82922 [CrossRef]
19. Costa, A.; Henriques, J.; Alarcão, V.; Madeira, T.; Virgolino, A.; Henriques, A.; Feteira-Santos, R.; Polley, M.; Arriaga, M Nogueira, P. Social prescribing for older adults in mainland Portugal: Perceptions and future prospects. *Prev. Med. Rep.* **202** *39*, 102652. [CrossRef]
20. Muhl, C.; Mulligan, K.; Bayoumi, I.; Ashcroft, R.; Godfrey, C. Establishing internationally accepted conceptual and operation definitions of social prescribing through expert consensus: A Delphi study. *BMJ Open* **2023**, *13*, e070184. [CrossRef]
21. O'Rourke, H.M.; Collins, L.; Sidani, S. Interventions to address social connectedness and loneliness for older adults: A scopin review. *BMC Geriatr.* **2018**, *18*, 214. [CrossRef]
22. Rogers, W.A.; Mitzner, T.L. Envisioning the future for older adults: Autonomy, health, well-being, and social connectedness wit technology support. *Futures* **2017**, *87*, 133–139. [CrossRef] [PubMed]
23. Høst, D.; Hendriksen, C.; Borup, I. Older people's perception of and coping with falling, and their motivation for fall-preventio programmes. *Scand. J. Public Health* **2011**, *39*, 742–748. [CrossRef] [PubMed]
24. Park, Y.; Kim, S.R.; Seo, H.-J.; Cho, J. Health Literacy in Fall-Prevention Strategy: A Scoping Review. *Asian Nurs. Res.* **202** *18*, 532–544. [CrossRef] [PubMed]
25. Thomas, E.; Battaglia, G.; Patti, A.; Brusa, J.; Leonardi, V.; Palma, A.; Bellafiore, M. Physical activity programs for balance and fa prevention in elderly: A systematic review. *Medicine* **2019**, *98*, e16218. [CrossRef]
26. Percival, A.; Newton, C.; Mulligan, K.; Petrella, R.J.; Ashe, M.C. Systematic review of social prescribing and older adults: Wher to from here? *Fam. Med. Community Health* **2022**, *10* (Suppl. S1), e001829. [CrossRef]
27. The EuroQol Group. EuroQol-a new facility for the measurement of health-related quality of life. *Health Policy* **1990**, *16*, 199–20 [CrossRef]
28. Sullivan, G.M.; Artino, A.R., Jr. Analyzing and interpreting data from Likert-type scales. *J. Grad. Med. Educ.* **2013**, *5*, 541 [CrossRef]
29. Warmoth, K.; Lang, I.A.; Phoenix, C.; Abraham, C.; Andrew, M.K.; Hubbard, R.E.; Tarrant, M. 'Thinking you're old and frail': A qualitative study of frailty in older adults. *Ageing Soc.* **2016**, *36*, 1483–1500. [CrossRef]
30. Alfaro Hudak, K.M.; Adibah, N.; Cutroneo, E.; Liotta, M.; Sanghera, A.; Weeks-Gariepy, T.; Strunz, E.; Rein, D.B. Older adults knowledge and perception of fall risk and prevention: A scoping review. *Age Ageing* **2023**, *52*, afad220. [CrossRef]
31. Burgon, C.; Darby, J.; Pollock, K.; Van Der Wardt, V.; Peach, T.; Beck, L.; Logan, P.; Harwood, R.H. Perspectives of healthcare professionals in England on falls interventions for people with dementia: A qualitative interview study. *BMJ Open* **2019**, *9*, e025702 [CrossRef]
32. Äijö, M.; Clifford, A.M.; Maguire, I.O. Preventing falls: Emphasizing education to support older person active ageing. In *Global Perspectives on Health Assessments for an Aging Population*; IGI Global: Hershey, PA, USA, 2023; pp. 137–155.
33. Khong, L.; Farringdon, F.; Hill, K.D.; Hill, A.-M. "We are all one together": Peer educators' views about falls prevention education for community-dwelling older adults-a qualitative study. *BMC Geriatr.* **2015**, *15*, 28. [CrossRef] [PubMed]
34. Howarth, M.; Griffiths, A.; Da Silva, A.; Green, R. Social prescribing: A 'natural'community-based solution. *Br. J. Community Nurs.* **2020**, *25*, 294–298. [CrossRef] [PubMed]
35. Prochaska, J.O.; DiClemente, C.C. Stages and processes of self-change of smoking: Toward an integrative model of change. *J. Consult. Clin. Psychol.* **1983**, *51*, 390. [CrossRef] [PubMed]
36. Rosenstock, I.M. The health belief model and preventive health behavior. *Health Educ. Monogr.* **1974**, *2*, 354–386. [CrossRef]

Johnston, Y.A.; Bergen, G.; Bauer, M.; Parker, E.M.; Wentworth, L.; McFadden, M.; Reome, C.; Garnett, M. Implementation of the stopping elderly accidents, deaths, and injuries initiative in primary care: An outcome evaluation. *Gerontologist* **2019**, *59*, 1182–1191. [CrossRef]
Wee, J.; Lysaght, R. Factors affecting measures of activities and participation in persons with mobility impairment. *Disabil. Rehabil.* **2009**, *31*, 1633–1642. [CrossRef]
Smith, M.L.; Ory, M.G. Multi-directional nature of falls among older adults: A rationale for prevention and management. *Front. Public Health* **2023**, *11*, 1117863. [CrossRef]
Wiseman, J.M.; Quatman, C.E.; Quatman-Yates, C.C. Examining Factors Influencing Older Adult Engagement in Fall Prevention: A Comparative Analysis Among Stakeholders. *J. Am. Geriatr. Soc.* **2025**, *73*, 1135–1143. [CrossRef]
WHO Team. *Healthy Ageing and Functional Ability [Internet]*; World Health Organization: Geneva, Switzerland, 2020. Available online: https://www.who.int/news-room/questions-and-answers/item/healthy-ageing-and-functional-ability (accessed on 13 October 2025).
Chesser, A.K.; Woods, N.K.; Reyes, J.; Rogers, N.L. Health literacy and older adults: Fall prevention and health literacy in a midwestern state. *J. Aging Res. Healthc.* **2018**, *2*, 31–40.
Fixsen, D.; Scott, V.; Blase, K.; Naoom, S.; Wagar, L. When evidence is not enough: The challenge of implementing fall prevention strategies. *J. Saf. Res.* **2011**, *42*, 419–422. [CrossRef]
Frick, K.D.; Kung, J.Y.; Parrish, J.M.; Narrett, M.J. Evaluating the cost-effectiveness of fall prevention programs that reduce fall-related hip fractures in older adults. *J. Am. Geriatr. Soc.* **2010**, *58*, 136–141. [CrossRef]

healthcare

MDPI

Article

Epidemiology of Falls Among Older Adults in Portugal: Analysis of Unintentional Injuries Reported by a National Emergency Surveillance System

Tatiana Alves [1,2,*], Susana Silva [1], Paula Braz [1], Maria Papadakaki [3], Carlos Aniceto [1], Ricardo Mexia [1] and Carlos Matias-Dias [1]

1 Epidemiology Department, National Institute of Health Doctor Ricardo Jorge, 1649 Lisbon, Portugal; susana.pereira@insa.min-saude.pt (S.S.); paula.braz@insa.min-saude.pt (P.B.); carlos.aniceto@insa.min-saude.pt (C.A.); ricardo.mexia@insa.min-saude.pt (R.M.); carlos.dias@insa.min-saude.pt (C.M.-D.)

2 Higher School of Health, Polytechnic Institute, 2914 Setubal, Portugal

3 Department of Social Work, Hellenic Mediterranean University, 71004 Heraklion, Greece; mpapadakaki@hmu.gr

* Correspondence: tatiana.alves@insa.min-saude.pt

Abstract: Background/Objectives: Falls occurring at home and during leisure time among elderly individuals represent a serious public health issue in Portugal and worldwide. These incidents have a significant impact on healthcare systems and social support structures, as well as the personal and family lives of the victims. There is also a recognized gap in awareness among older adults regarding fall prevention, particularly regarding environmental hazards, the need for home modifications, and the adoption of safety behaviors, including necessary adjustments in their home environments. The present study was developed to enhance our understanding of the circumstances in which falling occurs in elderly people. **Methods**: A cross-sectional epidemiological study was carried out, analyzing data collected through the national emergency-based injury surveillance system in 2023. **Results**: The proportion of falls increased across age groups, with 34.9% of total falls occurring in the group aged 85 and over. These differences were statistically significant ($p < 0.001$). In all age groups, falls were more frequent among women, representing between 63.6% and 69.0% of episodes. Approximately 65.9% of falls occurred at home. The likelihood of falling was higher among the oldest age group (85+) and in the home. **Conclusions**: The results of this study confirm that falls in elderly people tend to occur more frequently with advancing age, particularly in environments where the most time is spent. This study suggests that fall-prevention campaigns should be specifically targeted towards older females in the home environment, with particular consideration given to morning routines as part of the recommended interventions.

Keywords: injuries; home and leisure time; emergency department; hospitals; Portugal

1. Introduction

Falls are a global public health concern and represent the second leading cause of unintentional injury-related deaths, following road traffic accidents [1,2]. While falls can occur across all age groups, age is a well-established risk factor [3]. Understanding falls among older adults is particularly important within the global context of population ageing.

Falls are also a critical issue for emergency department (ED) teams, as they represent the leading cause of external injuries and account for approximately 24% of injury-related ED visits [4].

Numerous studies have shown that the frequency of falls increases with age and frailty. The risk of falling increases progressively in both men and women, across rural and urban populations, and among all ethnic groups [1].

Approximately 28–35% of individuals over the age of 65 experience at least one fall per year, with about half of them falling more frequently. Among those older than 70 and living in the community, the frequency increases to 32–42% [1].

Different factors have been identified in the occurrence of falls, usually classified as intrinsic and extrinsic. The intrinsic factors are usually related to chronic diseases, associated health conditions, sleep disorders, and polypharmacy. Due to their modifiable nature, environmental hazards—classified as extrinsic factors—are involved in 33–50% of falls [4]. Generally, it has been documented that most falls in the elderly occur indoors, namely, in the bathroom, bedroom, and kitchen. Elderly people tend to fall at home during routine activities.

In Portugal, demographic ageing is a well-documented reality, and this trend is expected to continue. This is driven not only by a decrease in the young and working-age population, but also by a steady increase in the number of older adults [5]. As a result, the incidence of falls are projected to increase, not only due to the growing elderly population, but also due to the age-related burden of comorbidities, polypharmacy, and frailty [4,6]. This evolving scenario could lead to a greater demand for emergency services [2].

According to data from the national injury surveillance system (EVITA), falls account for over 70% of injury mechanisms in home- and leisure-related incidents among older adults who present to emergency departments [7]. Furthermore, national data from 2023 show that approximately 11% of people aged 65 and older sought help in emergency departments due to a fall [8].

Several studies have highlighted the importance of fall prevention in older people, due to the significant impact falls can have on motor function, mobility, autonomy, and self-confidence [1,3]. These consequences often lead to mental health challenges, such as depression [6,7], anxiety [6,7], and social isolation [4].

Falls among older adults are often described in the literature as a multifactorial phenomenon, involving both intrinsic and extrinsic factors. The living environment plays a crucial role, as the characteristics and dynamics of falls vary depending on the context and location—particularly within the home or residential care settings [4,9].

Different factors have been reported to contribute to the occurrence of falls, which are usually classified as intrinsic and extrinsic. Intrinsic factors commonly include chronic diseases, comorbid health conditions, sleep disorders, and polypharmacy. On the other hand, extrinsic factors, such as environmental hazards, are modifiable and have been found to contribute to 33–50% of falls. These modifiable risks are often targeted in fall-prevention programs [4]. Research consistently shows that most falls among older adults occur indoors, especially in bathrooms, bedrooms, and kitchens, usually during routine daily activities.

Maintaining good health, autonomy, and independence for as long as possible is a major challenge for individuals and society alike, and has significant implications for national economic development. Nevertheless, the reality is that the later years of life are often marked by frailty and disability, conditions that are often preventable, especially in the case of falls.

Nurses play a critical role in fall prevention within the community setting. Although various nursing interventions have been developed to address this public health concern, understanding fall characteristics in specific contexts can support more tailored and effective strategies [10,11].

The aim of this study is to describe the characteristics of same-level and stair-related falls among individuals aged 65 and older, who accessed emergency services within Portugal's National Health Service in 2023. The study seeks to increase knowledge regarding the factors associated with falls in this population.

2. Materials and Methods

An observational, descriptive, cross-sectional epidemiological study was conducted, analyzing data from the national injury surveillance system (EVITA) for hospital emergency episodes in 2023 involving individuals aged 65 years and older in Portugal [12].

The EVITA system is a health observation tool that enables the monitoring of home and leisure accidents (HLA). The data were extracted from the Sistema Integrado de Informação Hospitalar (SONHO), the Integrated Hospital Information System responsible for generating, controlling, and invoicing administrative and clinical data, including patient history, diagnoses, and benefit information. SONHO facilitates the export of data for statistical indicators and supports clinical data sharing across hospitals and health centers that use this system (http://im.med.up.pt/si_saude/si_saude.html; https://aprendis.med.up.pt/index.php/SONHO, accessed on 1 May 2025). This system is used in more than 90% of health institutions within Portugal's National Health System (SNS), encompassing public and public—private partnership hospitals throughout all regions, ensuring extensive national coverage and representing the entire population.

A descriptive analysis (counts) was carried out based on variables including age group, sex, day of the week, time of the accident, place of occurrence, and discharge destination. Bivariate analysis was performed using Pearson's chi-squared test with a significance level set at 5%. For the inferential analysis, a logistic regression model was used and the results were presented as adjusted odds ratios (ORs) with 95% confidence intervals. The analysis was performed using the R Statistical Computing Environment program (R version 4.1.2) [13].

3. Results

This study analyzed the 35,312 emergency department admissions resulting from same-level and stair-related falls among older adults, as recorded in the national injury surveillance system (EVITA). An overall increase in the proportion of falls was observed across all age groups, with 34.9% of all falls occurring in individuals aged 85 and older.

When examining fall episodes by age and sex, falls were more frequent among women in all age groups, accounting for between 63.6% and 69.0% of cases. These differences were statistically significant ($p < 0.001$) (Table 1).

The timing of falls varied throughout the day, with the majority occurring during the morning and afternoon, between 09:00 a.m. and 17:00 p.m. This timeframe accounted for 52.3% of falls in the 85 and older age group and 55.5% in the 75–79 age group. Sunday had the lowest number of fall-related emergency department admissions across all age groups, although no statistically significant association was found between the day of the week and the age group.

Falls occurred in a variety of settings, with the home being the most common location (22,535 cases; 65.9%). Notably, the proportion of falls occurring at home increased with age, from 64.4% in the 65–74 age group to 68.9% in the 75–84 years. In the 65–74 age group, the most frequent fall locations after the home were transport areas (14.6%) and outdoor spaces (11.4%). In the 85 and. older age group, the second most common location was institutional settings (24.9%), with more than 80% of these falls occurring in residential or nursing homes.

Regarding discharge outcomes, the proportion of fall-related cases resulting in hospital admission increased with age, from 8.7% in the 65–74 age group to 18.7% in those aged 85 and over. Conversely, the proportion of cases that did not require further medical consultation, either in primary care or in hospital, decreased with age, from 49.0% in the 65–74 group to 43.4% in the 85 and over group.

Table 1. Distribution of fall episodes in people aged 65 and over, by sex, day of the week, time of accident, place of occurrence, and discharge destination (EVITA, 2023).

	Age Group						
	65–74		**75–84**		**≥85**		
	n	%	n	%	n	%	*p*-Value [1]
otal	9916	28.1	13,076	37.0	12,320	34.9	
ex							<0.001
ɪale	3610	36.4	4299	32.9	3825	31.0	
emale	6306	63.6	8777	67.1	8495	69.0	
Veek day							0.392
unday	1356	13.7	1783	13.6	1689	13.7	
ɅIonday	1383	13.9	1991	15.2	1839	14.9	
ʼuesday	1418	14.3	1872	14.3	1750	14.2	
Vednesday	1423	14.4	1843	14.1	1812	14.7	
ʼhursday	1405	14.2	1851	14.2	1726	14.0	
ʼriday	1481	14.9	1834	14.0	1733	14.1	
ɜunday	1450	14.6	1902	14.5	1771	14.4	
Accident time							<0.001
)0:00–08:59	1230	12.4	1934	14.8	2413	19.6	
09:00–16:59	5444	54.9	7261	55.5	6440	52.3	
17:00–24:59	3242	32.7	3881	29.7	3467	28.1	
Occurrence place							<0.001
Home	6123	64.4	8695	68.9	7717	64.1	
Outdoor spaces	1083	11.4	1046	8.3	509	4.2	
Transport area	1387	14.6	1257	10.0	640	5.3	
Trade area	180	1.9	184	1.5	78	0.6	
Institutional area	415	4.4	1178	9.3	2998	24.9	
Country area	320	3.4	266	2.1	100	0.8	
Destination after discharge							<0.001
Abandonment	282	2.8	234	1.8	159	1.3	
Unreferenced exterior	4850	49.0	6068	46.5	5384	43.8	
Referenced	3496	35.3	4625	35.4	3946	32.1	
Hospitalization	857	8.7	1598	12.2	1598	18.7	
Transferred another hospital	221	2.2	279	2.1	257	2.1	
Decease	5	0.1	13	0.1	24	0.2	
Other	186	1.9	233	1.8	218	1.8	

[1] Pearson's Chi-square test.

To examine the association between fall occurrence and factors such as sex, age group and place of occurrence, a logistic regression model was applied.

Regarding sex, the analysis showed that the odds of fall-related emergency department visits among older adults in Portugal during the 2023 year were 2.47 times higher in females than in males, a statistically significant finding (OR = 2.47; 95% [2.33, 2.62]) (Figure 1). In terms of age, individuals aged 85 and over had 4.47 times higher odds of experiencing a fall resulting in ED visit compared to those aged 65–74 year (OR = 4.47; 95% [4.10, 4.87]) a statistically significant result. Similarly, individuals in the 75–84 age group had higher odds of falls compared to the 65–64 age group (OR = 2.24, 95% [2.10, 2.38]).

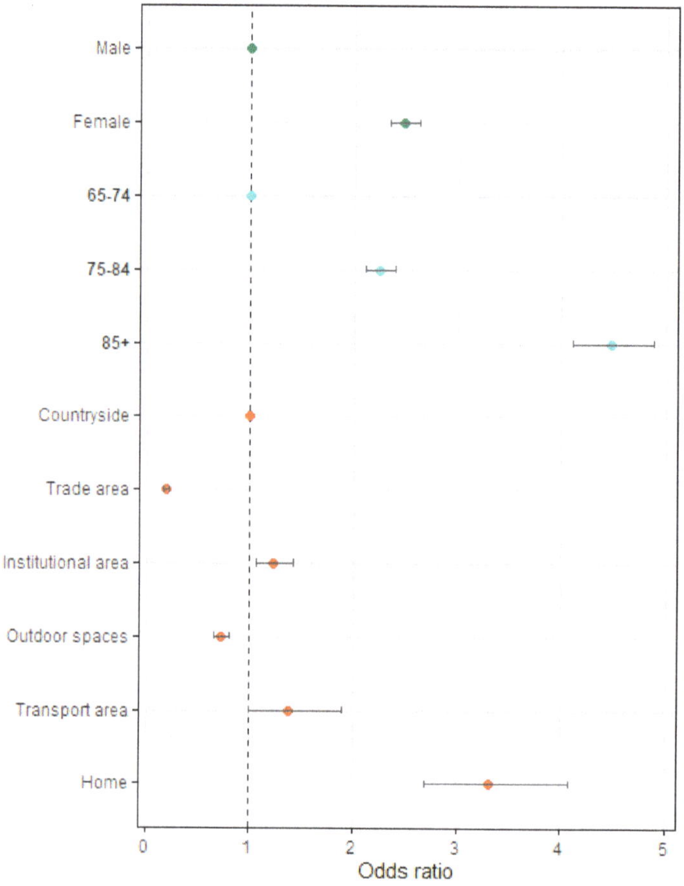

Figure 1. Adjusted odds ratio falls attended at the hospital emergency department, in the elderly people, in Portugal during the 2023 year by sex, age group and place of occurrence.

With respect to the place of occurrence, the odds of experiencing a fall at home were 3.31 times higher than in countryside settings, a statistically significant difference (OR = 3.31, 95% [2.69, 4.07]). Additionally, falls occurring in institutional settings were 1.23 times more likely than those occurring in the countryside (OR = 1.23; 95% CI [1.06, 1.42]). In contrast, falls that occurred in outdoor spaces (OR = 0.72; 95% CI [0.65, 0.79]) and in commercial areas (OR = 0.19; 95% CI [0.17, 0.22]) were significantly less likely compared with falls in countryside settings.

4. Discussion

Falls among elderly individuals represent a significant public health concern, given their high frequency, impact on healthcare utilization, and their role as a leading cause of hospital emergency departments visits.

In the population aged 65 years and over, falls emerged as the most common mechanism of injury. This study revealed an age-related increase in the proportion of falls, aligning with international findings that identify falls as the primary cause of emergency department admissions for unintentional injuries among the elderly [6,7,14–18].

The literature consistently underscores that while falls are a multifactorial phenomenon, age is one of the most frequently cited biological risk factors. Several studies have highlighted the role of aging in functional decline, leading to increased frailty and a higher likelihood of falling [3,4,16–18].

As observed in Portugal and other countries, women are more frequently affected by falls than men [16,19]. Various biological conditions associated with the female sex, including musculoskeletal disorders, are thought to contribute to this higher susceptibility to falls [4,10,17].

Regarding the timing of falls, this study found that they occurred most often toward the end of the week and during daily hours, which seems to be linked to the daily routines and activities of older adults. This pattern aligns with findings from other national and international studies [2,16,17]. However, a contrasting study conducted in Turkey reported no significant variation in fall incidence based on the time of day [7].

We found older adults requiring hospitalization as a result of a fall tended to be in the oldest age groups. This corroborates previous research indicating that increased age is associated with more severe injuries and longer hospital stays [4,20,21]. These findings highlight the need for health services, particularly nursing teams, in order to understand the implications of falls and plan interventions aimed at secondary and tertiary prevention in ageing populations.

Given their close interactions with patients, nurses—alongside other healthcare professionals such as physicians, pharmacists, physiotherapists, and occupational therapists—should play a key role in fall prevention. They need to be aware of the dimensions and characteristics of falls, recognize that older adults are at higher risk, and identify specific contributing factors. Working within an interdisciplinary team, nurses can contribute to implementing strategies and interventions aimed at modifying fall risk factors and improving safety in this vulnerable population [11,22]. Additionally, in the context of home hospitalization, nurses play a crucial role in educating older adults and their families about personalized measures to prevent falls. They consider the unique features of each residence and the individual's clinical conditions, providing ongoing monitoring to ensure safety [23,24].

The regression analysis revealed that being female and of an advanced age were independently associated with an increased risk of falls. These results are in line with other studies indicating out that being female is a risk factor for falls [25]. In comparison with males, females typically have lower muscle mass and weaker musculoskeletal systems [26]. Our study is also aligned with other studies showing that older adults are at a substantially greater risk for falls compared with younger adults [2].

The setting in which falls occur have also been increasingly studied, and several studies have shown that falls in older individuals predominantly occur at home and in institutional settings, similar to our observations in this study. Conversely, fewer falls occur in outdoor or public areas, possibly due to decreased mobility and activity levels among older adults, which reduce their exposure to these environments. Nonetheless, the literature emphasizes the importance of assessing and eliminating hazards in all settings to reduce environmental risks that contribute to falls [4,9,16,18].

While acknowledging the contributions of this study, it is crucial to recognize the inherent limitations that may influence the interpretation of its findings. The analysis focused exclusively on falls among individuals aged 65 and older who received emergency treatment at hospitals within Portugal's National Health Service. This approach may overlook less serious falls treated outside hospital settings or those that did not require medical attention, suggesting that the true incidence and impact of falls among older adults may be significantly underestimated. This raises questions regarding the thoroughness and precision of the surveillance data, as minor falls—despite being less severe—can still have significant consequences for health and well-being.

Moreover, the reliance on data collected from hospital admissions reported through the EVITA system, while methodologically standardized and in alignment with European injury surveillance protocols, limits generalizability to the broader older adult population. It presumes that documented cases are entirely representative; however, it overlooks individuals who fall and do not seek hospital treatment or those who receive care in other healthcare environments, resulting in an inherent selection bias. This underscores the need to interpret these findings within the context of the population's healthcare-seeking patterns and the system's ability to record all pertinent incidents.

On the other hand, a major strength of this study is its methodical data collection and adherence to a standardized European framework, which enhances the reliability and comparability of the findings across regions. This methodological rigor provides a strong foundation for guiding targeted interventions; however, the results should be viewed with an understanding of their limitations and potential gaps. Recognizing these limitations highlights the necessity for broader, multisource data collection methods to clarify the true extent of fall-related injuries in older adults, and to develop more effective preventative strategies.

5. Conclusions

The proportion of falls increased across all age groups. The likelihood of falling was higher among older individuals, women, those living at home, and residents in elderly care facilities.

As shown in the literature, there is a pressing need to deepen our understanding of the factors associated with falls in older adults, especially in the context of current demographic trends and population aging. Ongoing research in this area is essential, as it supports the development of targeted fall-prevention programs and informs preparedness across various levels of healthcare.

This study highlights the importance of addressing falls among older adults as a critical issue linked to population ageing. It also highlights the need for increased awareness and engagement among those who play a vital role in their lives, such as family members, caregivers, nurses, and other health professionals. In particular, this study suggests that fall-prevention campaigns should be targeted specifically towards older females in home settings, and recommendations including morning daily routines should be considered. Also, these findings contribute to fall surveillance systems by drawing attention to variables that need further study.

Author Contributions: Conceptualization, T.A. and S.S.; methodology, T.A., S.S. and C.M.-D.; software, S.S.; validation, P.B., S.S. and C.M.-D.; formal analysis, S.S.; investigation, T.A.; resources, R.M.; data curation, S.S.; writing—original draft preparation, T.A.; writing—C.A., P.B. and T.A.; and editing, C.A.; visualization, M.P.; supervision, C.M.-D.; project administration, C.M.-D. All authors have read and agreed to the published version of the manuscript.

Funding: This research received no external funding.

Institutional Review Board Statement: The study was conducted in accordance with the Declaration of Helsinki, and approved by the National Data Protection Commission (authorization n° 6807/2018, approval date: 22 May 2018).

Informed Consent Statement: Verbal informed consent was obtained from the participants. Verbal consent was obtained rather than written given the impossibility of obtaining it due to context of the place where consent is collected. This study does not involve identifiable persons. The important public interest of this study has been recognized.

Data Availability Statement: The original contributions presented in this study are included in the article. Further inquiries can be directed to the corresponding author.

Acknowledgments: The authors thank the Epidemiology Department Observation Unit of the National Institute of Health Doctor Ricardo Jorge for its support.

Conflicts of Interest: The authors declare no conflicts of interest. The funders had no role in the design of the study; in the collection, analyses, or interpretation of data; in the writing of the manuscript; or in the decision to publish the results.

Abbreviations

The following abbreviations are used in this manuscript:

EVITA	Portugal injury surveillance system
HLA	Home and Leisure Accidents
SONHO	Integrated Hospital Information System

eferences

World Health Organization. *Falls*; WHO: Geneva, Switzerland, 2021.
Cox, S.; Roggenkamp, R.; Bernard, S.; Smith, K. The epidemiology of elderly falls attended by emergency medical services in Victoria, Australia. *Injury* **2018**, *49*, 1712–1719. [CrossRef] [PubMed]
Ganz, D.A.; Latham, N.K. Prevention of Falls in Community-Dwelling Older Adults. *N. Engl. J. Med.* **2020**, *382*, 734–743. [CrossRef] [PubMed]
Akyol, A.D. Falls in the elderly: What can be done? *Int. Nurs. Rev.* **2007**, *54*, 191–196. [CrossRef] [PubMed]
de Estatística, I.N. *As Pessoas: 2022*; INE: Lisbon, Portugal, 2022; ISBN 978-989-25-0662-3.
Currie, L.M. Fall and injury prevention. In *Patient Safety and Quality: An Evidence-Based Handbook for Nurses*; Agency for Healthcare Research and Quality: Rockville, MD, USA, 2008.
Alves, T. Acidentes domésticos e de lazer ocorridos em pessoas com 65 e mais anos durante a pandemia da COVID-19: Comparação entre 2019 e 2020. *Bol. EpidemiolóGico Obs.* **2021**, *10*, 62–66.
SPMS. Dashboard BI-Hospitalar. Available online: https://bi-hospitalar.spms.min-saude.pt/ (accessed on 10 April 2024).
Lewis, S.R.; Griffin, X.L. Preventing falls in older people: The evidence for environmental interventions and why history matters. *Cochrane Database Syst. Rev.* **2023**, *2023*, ED000162. [CrossRef] [PubMed]
). Almeida, A.M.G.d. *Funcionalidade e Vulnerabilidade em Pessoas Idosas*; Universidade Católica Portuguesa: Lisboa, Portugal, 2017.
1. Takase, M. Falls as the result of interplay between nurses, patient and the environment: Using text-mining to uncover how and why falls happen. *Int. J. Nurs. Sci.* **2022**, *10*, 30–37. [CrossRef] [PubMed]
2. Alves, T.; Silva, S.; Rodrigues, E.; Braz, P.; Mexia, R.; Neto, M.; Matias Dias, C. *EVITA Epidemiologia e Vigilância dos Traumatismos e Acidentes: Relatório 2021*; INSA: Lisboa, Portugal, 2022. Available online: http://hdl.handle.net/10400.18/9173 (accessed on 10 April 2024).
3. R Core Team. *R: A Language and Environment for Statistical Computing*; R Foundation for Statistical Computing: Vienna, Austria, 2021; Available online: https://www.R-project.org/ (accessed on 10 April 2024).
4. Montero-Odasso, M.M.; Kamkar, N.; Pieruccini-Faria, F.; Osman, A.; Sarquis-Adamson, Y.; Close, J.; Hogan, D.B.; Hunter, S.W.; Kenny, R.A.; Lipsitz, L.A.; et al. Evaluation of clinical practice guidelines on fall prevention and management for older adults: A systematic review. *JAMA Netw* **2021**, *4*, e2138911. [CrossRef] [PubMed]
5. National Institute for Health and Care Excellence. *Surveillance of Falls in Older People: Assessing Risk and Prevention (NICEGuidelineCG161)*; National Institute for Health and Care Excellence: London, UK, 2019.
.6. O'Keeffe, A.; O'Grady, S.; Cronin, F.; Dolan, C.; O'Hea, A.; O'Shea, K.L.; Naughton, C. Evaluation of an emergency department falls pathway for older people: A patient chart review. *Int. Emerg. Nurs.* **2020**, *51*, 100869. [CrossRef] [PubMed]
17. Rubenstein, L.Z. Falls in older people: Epidemiology, risk factors and strategies for prevention. *Age Ageing* **2006**, *35* (Suppl. 2), ii37–ii41. [CrossRef] [PubMed]
18. Tripathy, N.K.; Jagnoor, J.; Patro, B.K.; Dhillon, M.S.; Kumar, R. Epidemiology of falls among older adults: A cross sectional study from Chandigarh. *Injury* **2015**, *46*, 1801–1805. [CrossRef] [PubMed]

19. Boyé, N.D.; Mattace-Raso, F.U.; Van der Velde, N.; Van Lieshout, E.M.; De Vries, O.J.; Hartholt, K.A.; Kerver, A.J.; Bruijninc M.M.; Van der Cammen, T.J.; Patka, P.; et al. Circumstances leading to injuriou fall in older men and women in Netherlan *Injury* **2014**, *45*, 1224–1230. [CrossRef] [PubMed]
20. Scuffham, P.; Chaplin, S.; Legood, R. Incidence and costs of unintentional falls in older people in the United Kingdom. *J. Epidem Community Heal.* **2003**, *57*, 740–744. [CrossRef] [PubMed]
21. Ambrose, A.F.; Paul, G.; Hausdorff, J.M. Risk factors for falls among older adults: A review of the literature. *Maturitas* **2013**, 51–61. [CrossRef] [PubMed]
22. Horta, R.d.S.T. Falls prevention in older people and the role of nursing. *Br. J. Community Nurs.* **2024**, *29*, 335–339. [CrossR [PubMed]
23. Andrade, A.M.; Silva, K.L.; Seixas, C.T.; Braga, P.P. Nursing practice in home care: An integrative literature review. *Rev. Br Enferm.* **2017**, *70*, 210–219. [CrossRef] [PubMed]
24. Minardi, R.; Cotta, M.; Morales Suárez-Varela, M.; Llopis González, A.; Sette, J.; Filho, C.; Real, E.R.; Antonio, J.; Ricós, D. hospitalización domiciliaria: Antecedentes, situación actual y perspectivas Informe especial. *Rev. Panam. De Salud Pública* **20** *10*, 45–55. Available online: www.scielo.org (accessed on 10 April 2024).
25. Sotoudeh, G.R.; Mohammadi, R.; Mosallanezhad, Z.; Viitasara, E.; Soares, J.J. The prevalence, circumstances and consequences unintentional falls among elderly Iranians: A population study. *Arch. Gerontol. Geriatr.* **2018**, *79*, 123–130. [CrossRef] [PubMed
26. Benichou, O.; Lord, S.R. *Rationale for Strengthening Muscle to Prevent Falls and Fractures: A Review of the Evidence*; Springer Ne York LLC.: New York, NY, USA, 2016. [CrossRef]

healthcare

MDPI

icle

ne-Year Changes in Depressive Symptoms and Cognitive ınction Among Brazilian Older Adults Attending Primary Care

nanda Maria Silva Rivoli [1], Antonio Pedro Gabriel Monteiro Galhardo [1], Giancarlo Lucchetti [2], ia Abreu Esper [1], Yan Lyncon Ribeiro [1], Gerson de Souza Santos [3], Helena José [4,5,6], Luís Sousa [4,6,7], Gail Low [8] 1 Luciano Magalhães Vitorino [1,*]

1 Faculty of Medicine of Itajubá, Itajubá 37502-138, MG, Brazil; ferivoli@gmail.com (F.M.S.R.); antoniopedrofmit@gmail.com (A.P.G.M.G.); liziaaesper@hotmail.com (L.A.E.); yan.obras2018@gmail.com (Y.L.R.)
2 School of Medicine, Federal University of Juiz de Fora (UFJF), Juiz de Fora 36038-330, MG, Brazil; g.lucchetti@yahoo.com.br
3 Department of Medicine, Centro Universitário Ages, Paripiranga 48430-000, BA, Brazil; gerson.s.santos@ages.edu.br
4 Atlântica School of Health, 2730-036 Barcarena, Portugal; hjose@uatlantica.pt (H.J.); luismmsousa@gmail.com (L.S.)
5 Health Sciences Research Unit: Nursing (UICISA: E), Nursing School of Coimbra, 3004-011 Coimbra, Portugal
6 RISE-Health, Faculty of Medicine, University of Porto, 4200-319 Porto, Portugal
7 Comprehensive Health Research Centre, University of Évora, 7000-801 Évora, Portugal
8 Faculty of Nursing, MacEwan University, Edmonton, AB T5J 4S2, Canada; lowg4@macewan.ca
* Correspondence: lucianoenf@yahoo.com.br; Tel.: +55-(35)-988008269

Abstract: Background: Aging is a global phenomenon closely associated with changes in cognitive function and mental health. These conditions substantially burden public health systems and adversely affect the quality of life of older adults. This study aimed to examine changes in depressive symptoms and cognitive function over a 12-month follow-up period in a cohort of Brazilian older adults attending primary care. **Methods**: This observational longitudinal study included a randomized sample of individuals aged ≥60 years residing in São Paulo, Brazil, and registered at a Primary Healthcare Unit (PHU). Data collection involved administering a sociodemographic and health questionnaire along with two validated instruments: the Geriatric Depression Scale-15 (GDS-15) and the Mini-Mental State Examination (MMSE). Linear regression models were used for the analyses. **Results**: A total of 368 older adults were included, with 63% being men and a mean age of 74.65 years. After one year, depressive symptoms showed a notable increase, with the mean GDS-15 score rising from 5.97 to 7.48 (Cohen-d = 0.542). Likewise, there was a decrease in the mean MMSE score ranging from 19.11 to 18.88 (Cohen-d = 0.216). Adjusted regression analyses revealed that depressive symptoms at baseline (B = 0.696; $p = 0.048$; $R^2 = 0.19$) and cognitive function at baseline (B = 0.444; $p < 0.001$; $R^2 = 0.26$) were predictive of their respective deteriorations over the follow-up period. **Conclusions**: Depressive symptoms and cognitive decline place a significant burden on public health systems in aging societies. These findings underscore the importance of continuous monitoring and early intervention strategies to mitigate their impact and enhance the quality of life for older adults.

Keywords: aging; depression; cognitive dysfunction; geriatric psychiatry; longitudinal studies

1. Introduction

The global demographic shift toward population aging carries substantial implications for public health systems worldwide [1]. In Brazil, approximately 14.7% of the population is aged 60 years or older. This proportion is projected to reach 64 million individuals by 2050 [1,2]. In comparison, 16.8% of the U.S. population and 28.4% of Japan's population are already aged 65 or older [2]. These demographic dynamics pose complex challenges to healthcare systems, especially regarding the management of chronic conditions, geriatric syndromes, and neuropsychiatric disorders such as late-life depression and cognitive impairment. Such conditions markedly impair functional independence and contribute to escalating healthcare expenditures [3,4].

Depression is among the most prevalent mental health conditions affecting older adults, with a global prevalence of 28.4%. Its frequency varies across regions, influenced by cultural and socioeconomic factors that shape the onset and progression of symptoms [5,6]. Similarly, cognitive decline represents another major concern, impacting 21.2% of older adults in long-term care facilities globally [6].

Evidence suggests both conditions frequently co-occur, reinforcing each other in a cycle that exacerbates both mental and cognitive health. Proposed underlying mechanisms include neuroinflammation, dysregulation of the hypothalamic–pituitary–adrenal (HPA) axis, and cerebrovascular dysfunction, which may jointly contribute to this bidirectional relationship [7]. Studies conducted in high-income countries indicate that depressive symptoms and cognitive decline become markedly more prevalent after the age of 75 [7,8].

In Brazil, depressive symptoms and cognitive decline present growing public health challenges, with national data indicating a rising prevalence, particularly among low-income and underserved populations [9,10]. Depressive disorders have become significant contributors to disability-adjusted life years (DALYs) in the country, with rates steadily increasing since 1990 [10].

Despite this, there remains a notable scarcity of longitudinal studies examining the trajectory of depressive symptoms and cognitive function in Brazil. Existing research is predominantly cross-sectional and often overlooks cultural and socioeconomic factors. Additionally, studies focusing on older adults utilizing primary healthcare services—an integral component of Brazil's healthcare system—are limited. Primary care settings are particularly relevant due to their accessibility, high patient volume, and potential for early identification and intervention. The scarcity of longitudinal studies hinders a comprehensive understanding of the relationship between depressive symptoms and cognitive decline in older adults. Although such studies allow for the observation of temporal changes, the specific influence of clinical and demographic factors on the progression of these conditions often remains underexplored. Evidence generated through longitudinal designs can still support the development of targeted community-based screening strategies, interventions, and policies [11].

Addressing these gaps is vital for improving both clinical practice and healthcare delivery. Depressive symptoms and cognitive decline significantly impair older adults' functionality and increase their reliance on healthcare services [12]. These conditions are often underdiagnosed in primary care, resulting in delayed treatment and missed opportunities for prevention [13].

To address these issues, this study aims to examine changes in depressive symptoms and cognitive function over a 12-month follow-up period in a cohort of Brazilian older adults attending primary care. Understanding their natural course may inform timely identification and early, targeted intervention among at-risk older adults [13]. The findings from this study may inform broader healthcare strategies by supporting the development of community-based interventions and guiding policy initiatives aimed at promoting healthy aging.

2. Materials and Methods

2.1. Study Design

This was an observational, longitudinal study (12-month follow-up), conducted among older adults (≥60 years) residing in São Paulo, Brazil. The study was conducted between 2018 and 2019 and was approved by the Research Ethics Committee of the São Paulo Municipal Health Department (approval number 2.961.352). All participants provided written informed consent before data collection at both baseline and follow-up. The study adhered to the ethical principles outlined in the Declaration of Helsinki.

2.2. Participants and Eligibility Criteria

A total of 400 older adults (aged ≥60 years) registered at the Marcus Wolosker Belenzinho Primary Healthcare Unit (PHU) in São Paulo were recruited at baseline. This PHU is part of the Unified Health System (Sistema Único de Saúde, SUS), which serves as the primary point of entry for healthcare services. The PHU is situated within an area that, in 2019, was home to some 40,000 persons, among whom 11% were aged 60 years or older. The SUS aims to ensure that primary healthcare facilities like this one address around 80% of the healthcare needs of older persons nationwide, as per the guidelines of Brazil's Ministry of Health.

2.3. Sample Size

Sample size calculations were performed using G*Power 3.1 software to ensure sufficient power for multivariate regression analyses. Assuming a small effect size ($f^2 = 0.10$), $\alpha = 0.05$, power $(1 - \beta) = 0.99$, and 7 predictors, a minimum sample size of 300 participants was required. To account for potential losses during follow-up, the sample size was increased by 25% [14], resulting in the recruitment of 400 participants. This final sample size is sufficient to perform robust statistical analyses should there be attrition.

2.4. Procedures at Baseline and Follow-Up

At baseline (Time 0), participants were randomly selected from PHU registries using patient identification numbers. Simple random sampling was applied using a computer-generated process in Microsoft Excel, in which patient record numbers were randomly drawn to compose the sample. Data collection was conducted between March and July 2018 during scheduled nursing consultations by a trained nurse with over 10 years of primary healthcare experience. The interviews lasted approximately 40 min and were conducted in private settings to ensure confidentiality. At this stage, participants were informed about the 12-month follow-up and received a scheduled return date. The same nurse who conducted the baseline assessments coordinated follow-up by reinforcing return appointments during routine care, which helped ensure participant retention.

At follow-up (Time 1), assessments were conducted between February and August 2019 using the same protocol. Participants were contacted via phone and scheduled for interviews at the PHU. The follow-up was completed with 368 participants, and all data were collected by the same experienced nurse to maintain consistency.

2.5. Measures

2.5.1. Independent Variables

Sociodemographic and health data, including age (years) and gender (male or female), were collected. So too were health-related variables: daily medication use (yes or no), daily number of medications, and the presence of chronic diseases ("Do you have any chronic conditions or diseases?" yes or no). Chronic conditions were defined as those lasting three months or longer, with examples provided, such as hypertension, diabetes, depression, heart disease, arthritis, and cancer. Additional variables included polypharmacy (use of five or more medications daily, yes or no) and a history of falls in the last 12 months (yes or no).

2.5.2. Dependent Variables

Depressive symptoms were assessed using the Geriatric Depression Scale-15 (GDS-15), a 15-item instrument validated in Brazilian Portuguese [15]. Scores range from 0 to 15, with higher scores indicating more severe depressive symptoms. The scale includes items such as "Do you feel that your life is empty?" with response options of Yes (1 point) or No (0 points), and "Do you feel happy most of the time?" with responses of Yes (0 points) or No (1 point). A total score of 6 or more suggests the presence of depressive symptoms. In the present sample, the GDS-15 demonstrated good internal consistency, with a Cronbach's alpha of 0.83.

The Mini-Mental State Examination (MMSE), a widely used tool for cognitive function screening in older adults, has been validated in Brazilian Portuguese [16]. Scores range from 0 to 30, with higher scores indicating better cognitive function. Items include "What is today's date?" under the domain of orientation to time, with responses scored as Correct (1 point) or Incorrect (0 points), and "Spell the word 'WORLD' backward", under attention and calculation, with scoring based on full correctness (1 point) or any errors (0 points). The MMSE assesses various domains, including memory, language, and visuospatial skills, with adjustments for educational differences in Brazilian populations [17,18]. In this study, MMSE cutoff scores followed the Brazilian context: 13 for illiterate individuals, 18 for those with up to 8 years of schooling, and 26 for individuals with more than 8 years of education [18]. For the MMSE, internal consistency analysis in the current sample yielded a Cronbach's alpha of 0.68, indicating an acceptable level of reliability.

2.6. *Statistical Analysis*

All statistical analyses were performed using SPSS version 26. Cases with missing data were excluded using complete-case analysis. No imputation methods were applied, as missingness was minimal and randomly distributed. Descriptive statistics were performed for continuous and categorical variables. Paired *t*-tests were used for within-group comparisons of continuous variables, and McNemar's test was applied for categorical variables. Effect sizes were calculated using Cohen's d, with thresholds for small ($d \leq 0.2$), medium ($d \approx 0.5$), and large ($d \geq 0.8$) effects [18]. To examine associations between depressive symptoms (GDS-15) and cognitive function (MMSE), simple and multiple linear regressions were used. Multivariate linear regression models adjusted for clinically relevant covariates ($p < 0.05$) included the number of medications, self-rated health, polypharmacy, and a history of falls. All analyses were performed with a significance level of $p < 0.05$ and a 95% confidence interval (CI).

3. Results

Of the 400 older adults recruited at baseline, 368 (92.0%) completed the 12-month follow-up. The majority were women (n = 293; 73.1%), with a mean age of 72.5 years (SD = 7.3). Most participants had low educational attainment, with 242 (60.6%) having ≤8 years of schooling and 89 (22.3%) reporting no formal education. Regarding marital status, 195 (48.9%) were married or cohabiting. A total of 253 participants (63.3%) reported monthly family income of up to twice the minimum wage. At baseline, 148 (36.9%) met the criteria for polypharmacy, 208 (51.9%) had multimorbidity (≥2 chronic conditions), and 139 (34.8%) reported at least one fall in the previous year. These characteristics are detailed in Table 1.

Table 1. Sociodemographic and health profiles of participants at baseline (T0) and 12-month follow-up (T1) [a].

Variables	2018 (n = 368)	2019 (n = 368)	*p*-Value
Age (M; SD)	74.65 (7.99)	75.36 (7.79)	0.058
Number of Medications	3.83 (2.02)	4.68 (1.65)	<0.001
	n (%)	n (%)	
Gender			
Male	232 (63.0)	233 (63.3)	>0.999
Female	136 (37.0)	135 (36.7)	
Self-Perceived Health			
Excellent	28 (7.60)	16 (4.35)	
Good	114 (30.97)	97 (26.38)	0.001
Fair	148 (40.22)	137 (37.23)	
Poor	78 (21.21)	118 (32.03)	
Chronic disease			
Yes	338 (91.84)	367 (99.72)	<0.001
No	30 (8.15)	1 (0.27)	
Polypharmacy (≥5 medications)			
Yes	136 (36.95)	247 (67.12)	<0.001
No	232 (63.05)	121 (32.88)	
History of Falls [b]			
Yes	251 (68.20)	367 (99.80)	<0.001
No	148 (31.80)	1 (0.20)	

[a] Older adults (n = 32) who participated at the baseline but not follow-up were excluded from this analysis. [b] in the 1st 12 months. SD: Standard Deviation.

Table 2 shows that scores on the Geriatric Depression Scale (GDS-15) increased significantly from 5.97 (SD = 2.91) to 7.48 (SD = 2.65) ($p < 0.001$), yielding a moderate effect size (d = 0.542). Concurrently, there was a slight (d = 0.216) but significant decline in Mini-Mental State Examination (MMSE) scores, from 19.88 (SD = 2.92) to 19.11 (SD = 2.97) ($p < 0.001$). Cognitive decline, while modest, was statistically significant.

Table 2. Comparison of depressive symptoms and cognitive function of participants (n = 368).

Variables	T0 (n = 368)	T1 (n = 368)	*p*-Value	Effect Size
Depressive Symptoms	Mean (SD)	Mean (SD)		
GDS-15	5.97 (2.91)	7.48 (2.65)	<0.001	0.542
Cognitive Function				
MMSE	19.88 (2.92)	19.11 (2.97)	<0.001	0.216

SD: Standard Deviation; GDS-15: Geriatric Depression Scale-15; MMSE: Mini-Mental State Examination.

In Table 3, the adjusted linear regression analysis revealed that higher levels of depressive symptoms at baseline were significantly associated with higher depressive symptom levels at 12 months (B = 0.696; $p = 0.048$). Similarly, lower cognitive function at baseline (Time 0) predicted greater cognitive decline one year later at Time 1 (B = 0.444; $p < 0.001$).

Table 3. Adjusted linear regression analyses of depressive symptoms and cognitive function at baseline (Time 0) and 12-month follow-up (Time 1).

Variables	B (SE)	Beta	*p*-Value	Adjusted R^2
GDS-15 *	0.123 (0.047)	0.135	<0.001	0.13
GDS-15 ** (Sociodemographic and Clinical)	0.696 (0.386)	0.110	0.048	0.19
MMSE *	0.465 (0.047)	0.457	<0.001	0.29
MMSE ** (Sociodemographic and Clinical)	0.444 (0.049)	0.437	<0.001	0.26

* GDS-15 and MMSE without adjustment; ** GDS-15 and MMSE adjusted for clinical variables (number of medications, self-perceived health, polypharmacy, history of falls). SE: Standard Error.

4. Discussion

This longitudinal study provides important insights into the progression of depressive symptoms and cognitive decline among older adults utilizing primary healthcare services in Brazil. Over a 12-month period, we observed a significant worsening of depressive symptoms, alongside a modest but statistically significant decline in cognitive function.

The observed increase in depressive symptoms, as measured by the GDS-15, aligns with prior studies highlighting a growing burden of emotional distress among older adults over time [19–21]. However, in our sample, we observed a moderate statistically significant increase in mean GDS-15 scores after one year.

We also found substantial increases in polypharmacy (from 36.95% to 67.12%), a factor known to exacerbate depressive symptoms [22,23]. Polypharmacy is commonly defined as the concurrent use of five or more medications, whereas excessive polypharmacy refers to the use of ten or more medications [24,25]. In older adults, polypharmacy has been associated with a significantly higher risk of depression, largely due to adverse drug interactions, side effects, and the cognitive burden of complex medication regimens [22].

Polypharmacy can be associated with multiple adversities, including dementia, enhanced symptoms of depression, and even death [26]. Robust evidence indicates that managing complex medication regimens may reduce social motivation and contribute to anxiety, particularly in later life [27–29]. We examined data over one year of time. Longer-term observations are warranted to further uncouple links between medication regimens and depressive symptoms.

Cognitive decline, assessed through the MMSE, was modest but statistically significant, corroborating findings from other longitudinal studies involving community-dwelling older adults [30,31]. Despite a small effect size, the steady decline in MMSE scores highlights the vulnerability of cognitive function in aging populations, especially in individuals with multimorbidity and polypharmacy [24,32–36].

Notably, the rise in polypharmacy and a history of falls likely further exacerbated cognitive decline [32,37,38]. Cognitive impairment is known to increase fall risks over time [33,39]. Polypharmacy is a double-edged sword with many ugly sides. Other pernicious companions include a slower gait [40], frequent hospital admissions, and non-beneficial medication prescribing [33]. A slower gait has enhanced some community-dwelling older persons' risk of falling for up to one year [41]. Less capacity to get out and about of one's own volition, albeit from falls or other traumas, and shrinking social circles can aggravate emotional distress in later life [28,29]. Some older people experiencing physically traumatic events report taking 10 or more medications a day [36]. Persistent complex regimens have put others at a significantly higher risk for fall-related injuries in both hospital and outpatient settings [25].

These findings reinforce the need for regular reviews of pharmacological regimens, focusing on therapeutic necessity and minimizing exposure to fall-risk-increasing drugs

(FRIDs) such as narcotics, diuretics, beta-blockers, and antipsychotics [25,34,39,42,43]. Cognitive impairment can complicate clinical assessment by masking or mimicking symptoms of other conditions, especially in individuals living with dementia [32]. Therefore, comprehensive evaluation and cautious deprescribing strategies are essential in this population.

Best practices for reducing opioids, benzodiazepines, and other FRIDs should include fall and depression-related risk education and transparent co-designed follow-up plans for patients and their families. Patients without family would benefit from a PHU advocate such as a Nurse Practitioner. Good deprescribing duly considers older persons' overall health and comfort [34,44].

Ultimately, older persons are the ones who have to live with the psychological impacts of medication regimens, day in and day out. Older persons residing in 20 different countries have reported that quality living is about being one's own health steward, both with clarity of mind and with healthcare practitioners knowing what they value and expect, and their immediate living environment [45]. This cannot be over-emphasized. In this study, as others point out [46], depressive symptoms and cognitive decline can and do co-exist in later life. Depression may impair cognitive processes, such as memory, attention, and executive function, while cognitive decline can exacerbate depressive symptoms by reducing independence and quality of life [47].

While this bidirectional relationship is well-recognized, the temporal sequence remains unclear. A meta-analysis of community-based cohort studies found that late-life depression nearly doubles the risk of developing dementia [48]. Additionally, psychosocial stressors—including perceived stress, social isolation, and low emotional support—have been independently associated with accelerated cognitive decline in older adults [49]. These findings reinforce the hypothesis of shared neurobiological mechanisms and highlight the need for integrated assessment and management strategies in primary care.

We implore healthcare practitioners to keep this vicious circle in mind early, at the forefront of co-decision-making and co-design of follow-up planning.

Another best practice is establishing a community of care wherein patients and practitioners steer the clinical decision-making rudders [50]. Shared decision-making and clarity of mind are ideal steadfast companions, while practitioner-devised complex drug regimens and lived cognitive impairment are not. Older people have long argued that having a stake in decision making is important [51]. This can entail exploring, early on, older persons' preferences for the number of medications and their perceived impacts and capacity to manage them.

These findings have important implications for clinical practice. The observed increase in depressive symptoms over 12 months underscores the need for the early identification and timely treatment of depression in older adults. Routine depression screening in primary care settings using validated tools like the GDS-15 should be a priority early on to enhance diagnostic accuracy [52]. Early interventions, including both pharmacological and non-pharmacological approaches such as cognitive-behavioral therapy and social engagement programs, are also recommended to keep depressive symptoms in tow. Primary care providers should incorporate tools like the MMSE or Mini-Cog into routine evaluations, particularly for patients with known risk factors such as polypharmacy and a history of falls [53,54].

Finally, the study highlights the urgent need for a multidisciplinary approach in primary care. Given the interconnected nature of depressive symptoms and cognitive decline, collaboration among geriatricians, psychologists, and primary care providers is essential. Comprehensive care models addressing both mental and physical health could improve outcomes for older adults while reducing long-term healthcare burdens [53].

Other essential practitioners helping older persons to co-design follow-up plans include pharmacists, nurse practitioners, and occupation therapists.

Despite its strengths, this study has several limitations. The sample was drawn from a single PHU in São Paulo, which may limit the generalizability of what we found. Additionally, while validated instruments (GDS-15 and MMSE) were used, the reliance on self-reported data for variables such as medication use and fall history may introduce recall bias. Although comorbidities and socioeconomic status were included as covariates in the regression models, their individual contributions to the outcomes were not examined in depth, representing a limitation of this study. Social determinants such as low income, limited access to health services, and reduced social support are known to negatively impact both mental health and cognitive trajectories in aging populations.

Integrating these contextual factors into prevention strategies is essential to reduce disparities and promote healthy aging in primary care settings. Although the study has important strengths, it did not account for several potentially relevant contextual factors, which may have influenced the outcomes. Future research should consider integrating objective measures and examining the influence of key social determinants—such as socioeconomic status, living environment, and access to adjunct therapies and programs—on the progression of depressive symptoms and cognitive decline. Expanding longitudinal studies to diverse settings would also enhance our understanding of these conditions and their broader implications.

5. Conclusions

This study demonstrates that depressive symptoms and cognitive decline are significant and interrelated challenges for older adults in primary care settings. The observed worsening of depressive symptoms and modest cognitive decline over 12 months underscores the importance of early detection and intervention.

Our findings advocate for routine screening and the early adoption of comprehensive and co-designed interventions to mitigate the impact of these conditions. Future research should focus on elucidating the mechanisms linking depressive symptoms and cognitive decline and evaluating the effectiveness of co-designated early intervention and follow-up plans. We can best uncouple these links within multi-disciplinary teams with older people helping to steer clinical decision-making rudders.

Author Contributions: Conceptualization, L.M.V. and G.d.S.S.; methodology, L.M.V. and G.d.S.S.; software, L.M.V.; validation, L.M.V., L.S., G.L. (Gail Low) and G.L. (Giancarlo Lucchetti); formal analysis, L.M.V.; investigation, L.M.V. and G.d.S.S.; data curation, L.M.V., G.L. (Gail Low) and G.L. (Giancarlo Lucchetti); writing—original draft preparation, F.M.S.R., A.P.G.M.G., L.A.E., L.S. and Y.L.R.; writing—review and editing, L.M.V., L.S., G.L. (Gail Low), H.J. and G.L. (Giancarlo Lucchetti); visualization, L.M.V., H.J., L.S., G.L. (Gail Low) and G.L. (Giancarlo Lucchetti); supervision, L.M.V.; project administration, L.M.V. All authors have read and agreed to the published version of the manuscript.

Funding: This research received no external funding.

Institutional Review Board Statement: The study was conducted in accordance with the Declaration of Helsinki and approved on 5 July 2023 by the Research Ethics Committee of the São Paulo Municipal Health Department (approval number 2.961.352).

Informed Consent Statement: Informed consent was obtained from all subjects involved in the study.

Data Availability Statement: Data will be available upon request (lucianoenf@yahoo.com.br).

Conflicts of Interest: The authors declare no conflicts of interest.

References

1. Dall, T.M.; Gallo, P.D.; Chakrabarti, R.; West, T.; Semilla, A.P.; Storm, M.V. An Aging Population and Growing Disease Burden Will Require a Large and Specialized Health Care Workforce by 2025. *Health Aff.* **2013**, *32*, 2013–2020. [CrossRef]
2. Tramujas Vasconcellos Neumann, L.; Albert, S.M. Aging in Brazil. *Gerontologist* **2018**, *58*, 611–617. [CrossRef]
3. Prince, M.J.; Wu, F.; Guo, Y.; Gutierrez Robledo, L.M.; O'Donnell, M.; Sullivan, R.; Yusuf, S. The Burden of Disease in Older People and Implications for Health Policy and Practice. *Lancet* **2015**, *385*, 549–562. [CrossRef]
4. GBD 2019 Dementia Forecasting Collaborators. Estimation of the Global Prevalence of Dementia in 2019 and Forecasted Prevalence in 2050: An Analysis for the Global Burden of Disease Study 2019. *Lancet Public Health* **2022**, *7*, e105–e125. [CrossRef]
5. Hu, T.; Zhao, X.; Wu, M.; Li, Z.; Luo, L.; Yang, C.; Yang, F. Prevalence of Depression in Older Adults: A Systematic Review and Meta-Analysis. *Psychiatry Res.* **2022**, *311*, 114511. [CrossRef]
6. Chen, P.; Cai, H.; Bai, W.; Zhang, Q.; Su, Z.; Tang, Y.-L.; Ungvari, G.S.; Ng, C.H.; Xiang, Y.-T. Global Prevalence of Mild Cognitive Impairment among Older Adults Living in Nursing Homes: A Meta-Analysis and Systematic Review of Epidemiological Surveys. *Transl. Psychiatry* **2023**, *13*, 88. [CrossRef]
7. Weyerer, S.; Eifflaender-Gorfer, S.; Wiese, B.; Luppa, M.; Pentzek, M.; Bickel, H.; Bachmann, C.; Scherer, M.; Maier, W.; Riedel-Heller, S.G. Incidence and Predictors of Depression in Non-Demented Primary Care Attenders Aged 75 Years and Older: Results from a 3-Year Follow-up Study. *Age Ageing* **2013**, *42*, 173–180. [CrossRef]
8. Borelli, W.V.; Zimmer, E.R.; Bieger, A.; Coelho, B.; Pascoal, T.A.; Chaves, M.L.F.; Amariglio, R.; Castilhos, R.M. Subjective Cognitive Decline in Brazil: Prevalence and Association with Dementia Modifiable Risk Factors in a Population-Based Study. *Alzheimer's Dement. Diagn. Assess. Dis. Monit.* **2022**, *14*, e12368. [CrossRef]
9. Zenebe, Y.; Akele, B.; W/Selassie, M.; Necho, M. Prevalence and Determinants of Depression among Old Age: A Systematic Review and Meta-Analysis. *Ann. Gen. Psychiatry* **2021**, *20*, 55. [CrossRef]
10. Bonadiman, C.S.C.; Malta, D.C.; de Azeredo Passos, V.M.; Naghavi, M.; Melo, A.P.S. Depressive Disorders in Brazil: Results from the Global Burden of Disease Study 2017. *Popul. Health Metr.* **2020**, *18* (Suppl. 1), 6. [CrossRef]
11. da Nóbrega, I.R.A.P.; Leal, M.C.C.; Marques, A.P.d.O.; Vieira, J.d.C.M. Fatores Associados à Depressão Em Idosos Institucionalizados: Revisão Integrativa. *Saúde Debate* **2015**, *39*, 536–550. [CrossRef]
12. García-Peña, C.; Espinel-Bermúdez, C.; Tella-Vega, P.; Pérez-Zepeda, M.U.; Gutiérrez-Robledo, L.M. Longitudinal Studies and Older Adults Cohorts. In *Aging Research—Methodological Issues*; García-Peña, C., Gutiérrez-Robledo, L.M., Pérez-Zepeda, M.U., Eds.; Springer International Publishing: Cham, Switzerland, 2018; pp. 95–113. [CrossRef]
13. Pereira, M.E.A.; Santos, G.d.S.; Almeida, C.R.d.; Nunes, K.C.S.; Silva, M.C.M.d.; José, H.; Sousa, L.; Vitorino, L.M. Association between Falls, Fear of Falling and Depressive Symptoms in Community-Dwelling Older Adults. *Healthcare* **2024**, *12*, 1638. [CrossRef]
14. Fewtrell, M.S.; Kennedy, K.; Singhal, A.; Martin, R.M.; Ness, A.; Hadders-Algra, M.; Koletzko, B.; Lucas, A. How much loss to follow-up is acceptable in long-term randomised trials and prospective studies? *Arch. Dis. Child.* **2008**, *93*, 458–461.
15. Paradela, E.M.P.; Lourenço, R.A.; Veras, R.P. Validação Da Escala de Depressão Geriátrica Em Um Ambulatório Geral. *Rev. Saúde Pública* **2005**, *39*, 918–923. [CrossRef]
16. Folstein, M.F.; Folstein, S.E.; McHugh, P.R. "Mini-Mental State". A Practical Method for Grading the Cognitive State of Patients for the Clinician. *J. Psychiatr. Res.* **1975**, *12*, 189–198. [CrossRef]
17. Laks, J.; Baptista, E.M.R.; Contino, A.L.B.; de Paula, E.O.; Engelhardt, E. Mini-Mental State Examination Norms in a Community-Dwelling Sample of Elderly with Low Schooling in Brazil. *Cad. Saúde Pública* **2007**, *23*, 315–319. [CrossRef]
18. Bertolucci, P.H.; Brucki, S.M.; Campacci, S.R.; Juliano, Y. The Mini-Mental State Examination in a General Population: Impact of Educational Status. *Arq. Neuropsiquiatr.* **1994**, *52*, 1–7.
19. Schaakxs, R.; Comijs, H.C.; Lamers, F.; Beekman, A.T.F.; Penninx, B.W.J.H. Age-Related Variability in the Presentation of Symptoms of Major Depressive Disorder. *Psychol. Med.* **2017**, *47*, 543–552. [CrossRef]
20. Wilder, M.E.; Kulie, P.; Jensen, C.; Levett, P.; Blanchard, J.; Dominguez, L.W.; Portela, M.; Srivastava, A.; Li, Y.; McCarthy, M.L. The Impact of Social Determinants of Health on Medication Adherence: A Systematic Review and Meta-Analysis. *J. Gen. Intern. Med.* **2021**, *36*, 1359–1370. [CrossRef]
21. Comijs, H.C.; Nieuwesteeg, J.; Kok, R.; van Marwijk, H.W.; van der Mast, R.C.; Naarding, P.; Voshaar, R.C.O.; Verhaak, P.; de Waal, M.W.; Stek, M.L. The Two-Year Course of Late-Life Depression; Results from the Netherlands Study of Depression in Older Persons. *BMC Psychiatry* **2015**, *15*, 20. [CrossRef]
22. Vitorino, L.M.; Lopes, J.; Souza Santos, G.; Oliveira, C.; Helena, J.; Sousa, L. Prevalence of Polypharmacy of Older People in a Large Brazilian Urban Center and its Associated Factors. *Int. J. Environ. Res. Public Health* **2023**, *20*, 5730. [CrossRef]
23. Livingston, G.; Huntley, J.; Liu, K.Y.; Costafreda, S.G.; Selbæk, G.; Alladi, S.; Ames, D.; Banerjee, S.; Burns, A.; Brayne, C.; et al. Dementia Prevention, Intervention, and Care: 2024 Report of the Lancet Standing Commission. *Lancet* **2024**, *404*, 572–628. [CrossRef]

24. Yu, X.; Qian, Y.; Zhang, Y.; Chen, Y.; Wang, M. Association between Polypharmacy and Cognitive Impairment in Older Adults Systematic Review and Meta-Analysis. *Geriatr. Nurs.* **2024**, *59*, 330–337. [CrossRef]
25. Xue, L.; Boudreau, R.M.; Donohue, J.M.; Zgibor, J.C.; Marcum, Z.A.; Costacou, T.; Newman, A.B.; Waters, T.M.; Strotmeyer, Persistent Polypharmacy and Fall Injury Risk: The Health, Aging and Body Composition Study. *BMC Geriatr.* **2021**, *21*, 7 [CrossRef]
26. Palapinyo, S.; Methaneethorn, J.; Leelakanok, N. Association between Polypharmacy and Depression: A Systematic Review a Meta-Analysis. *J. Pharm. Pract. Res.* **2021**, *51*, 280–299. [CrossRef]
27. Wiersema, C.; Oude Voshaar, R.C.; van den Brink, R.H.S.; Wouters, H.; Verhaak, P.; Comijs, H.C.; Jeuring, H.W. Determina and Consequences of Polypharmacy in Patients with a Depressive Disorder in Later Life. *Acta Psychiatr. Scand.* **2022**, *146*, 85– [CrossRef]
28. World Health Organization. WHO Launches Commission to Foster Social Connection. 2023. Available online: https://www.w int/news/item/15-11-2023-who-launches-commission-to-foster-social-connection (accessed on 3 March 2025).
29. Maese, E. Almost a Quarter of the World Feels Lonely. 2023. Available online: https://news.gallup.com/opinion/gallup/5126 /almost-quarter-world-feels-lonely.aspx (accessed on 3 March 2025).
30. Beekman, A.T.F.; Geerlings, S.W.; Deeg, D.J.H.; Smit, J.H.; Schoevers, R.S.; de Beurs, E.; Braam, A.W.; Penninx, B.W.J.H.; v Tilburg, W. The Natural History of Late-Life Depression: A 6-year prospective study in the community. *Arch. Gen. Psychiat* **2002**, *59*, 605. [CrossRef]
31. Chui, H.; Gerstorf, D.; Hoppmann, C.A.; Luszcz, M.A. Trajectories of Depressive Symptoms in Old Age: Integrating Ag Pathology-, and Mortality-Related Changes. *Psychol. Aging G* **2015**, *30*, 940–951. [CrossRef]
32. Zhao, M.; Chen, Z.; Xu, T.; Ping, F.; Tian, F. Global Prevalence of Polypharmacy and Potentially Inappropriate Medication Older Patients with Dementia: A Systematic Review and Meta-Analysis. *Front. Pharmacol.* **2023**, *14*, 1221069. [CrossRef]
33. Scheel, J.; Luttenberger, K.; Graessel, E.; Kratzer, A.; Donath, C. Predictors of Falls and Hospital Admissions in People wi Cognitive Impairment in Day-Care: Role of Multimorbidity, Polypharmacy, and Potentially Inappropriate Medication. *BM Geriatr.* **2022**, *22*, 682. [CrossRef]
34. Ie, K.; Chou, E.; Boyce, R.D.; Albert, S.M. Fall Risk-Increasing Drugs, Polypharmacy, and Falls among Low-Income Communit Dwelling Older Adults. *Innov. Aging* **2021**, *5*, igab001. [CrossRef]
35. Leelakanok, N.; D'Cunha, R.R. Association between Polypharmacy and Dementia—A Systematic Review and Metaanalysi *Aging Ment. Health* **2018**, *23*, 932–941. [CrossRef]
36. de Godoi Rezende Costa Molino, C.; Rübel, L.; Mantegazza, N.; Bischoff-Ferrari, H.A.; Freystaetter, G. Association of Polypha macy with Cognitive Impairment in Older Trauma Patients: A Cross-Sectional Study. *Eur. J. Hosp. Pharm.* **2023**, *31*, 428–43 [CrossRef]
37. Lovett, R.; Bonham, M.; Benavente, J.Y.; Hosseinian, Z.; Byrne, G.J.; Diaz, M.V.; Bass, M.; Yao, L.; Adin-Cristian, A.; Batio, S et al. Primary Care Detection of Cognitive Impairment Leveraging Health and Consumer Technologies in Underserved U Communities: Protocol for a Pragmatic Randomised Controlled Trial of the MyCog Paradigm. *BMJ Open* **2023**, *13*, e08010 [CrossRef]
38. Pettigrew, C.; Soldan, A. Defining Cognitive Reserve and Implications for Cognitive Aging. *Curr. Neurol. Neurosci. Rep.* **2019** *19*, 1. [CrossRef]
39. Zhang, X.; Jiao, J.; Guo, N.; Bo, H.; Xu, T.; Wu, X. Association of Polypharmacy with Falls among Older Chinese Inpatients: A Nationwide Cohort Study. *Geriatr. Gerontol. Int.* **2021**, *21*, 810–817. [CrossRef]
40. Watanabe, K.; Umegaki, H.; Sugimoto, T.; Fujisawa, C.; Komiya, H.; Nagae, M.; Yamada, Y.; Kuzuya, M.; Sakurai, T. Associations between Polypharmacy and Gait Speed according to Cognitive Impairment Status: Cross-Sectional Study in a Japanese Memory Clinic. *J. Alzheimer's Dis.* **2021**, *82*, 1115–1122. [CrossRef]
41. Adam, C.E.; Fitzpatrick, A.L.; Leary, C.S.; Hajat, A.; Ilango, S.D.; Park, C.; Phelan, E.A.; Semmens, E.O. Change in Gait Speed and Fall Risk among Community-Dwelling Older Adults with and without Mild Cognitive Impairment: A Retrospective Cohort Analysis. *BMC Geriatr.* **2023**, *23*, 328. [CrossRef]
42. Hoel, R.W.; Giddings Connolly, R.M.; Takahashi, P.Y. Polypharmacy Management in Older Patients. *Mayo Clin. Proc.* **2021**, *96*, 242–256. [CrossRef]
43. Sousa, L.; Tomás, J.; Severino, S.; Valido, S.; Santos, M.J.; José, H. Prevention of Falls in the Elderly: A Challenge in Patient Safety *Salud Sci. Technol.* **2024**, *4*, 1000. [CrossRef]
44. Bai, W.; Chen, P.; Cai, H.; Zhang, Q.; Su, Z.; Cheung, T.; Jackson, T.; Sha, S.; Xiang, Y.-T. Worldwide Prevalence of Mild Cognitive Impairment among Community Dwellers Aged 50 Years and Older: A Meta-Analysis and Systematic Review of Epidemiology Studies. *Age Ageing* **2022**, *51*, afac173. [CrossRef] [PubMed]
45. World Health Organization. WHOQOL: Measuring Quality of Life. 2025. Available online: https://www.who.int/tools/whoqol (accessed on 3 March 2025).

Steffens, D.C.; Manning, K.J.; Wu, R.; Grady, J.J. Effects of Longitudinal Changes in Neuroticism and Stress on Cognitive Decline. *Am. J. Geriatr. Psychiatry* **2023**, *31*, 171–179. [CrossRef] [PubMed]
Zhu, Y.; Li, C.; Xie, W.; Zhong, B.; Wu, Y.; Blumenthal, J.A. Trajectories of Depressive Symptoms and Subsequent Cognitive Decline in Older Adults: A Pooled Analysis of Two Longitudinal Cohorts. *Age Ageing* **2021**, *51*, afab191. [CrossRef]
Diniz, B.S.; Butters, M.A.; Albert, S.M.; Dew, M.A.; Reynolds, C.F., 3rd. Late-life depression and risk of vascular dementia and Alzheimer's disease: Systematic review and meta-analysis of community-based cohort studies. *Br. J. Psychiatry* **2013**, *202*, 329–335.
Turner, A.D.; James, B.D.; Capuano, A.W.; Aggarwal, N.T.; Barnes, L.L. Perceived Stress and Cognitive Decline in Different Cognitive Domains in a Cohort of Older African Americans. *Am. J. Geriatr. Psychiatry* **2017**, *25*, 25–34. [CrossRef]
Power, M.; Quinn, K.; Schmidt, S. Development of the WHOQOL-Old Module. *Qual. Life Res.* **2005**, *14*, 2197–2214. [CrossRef]
World Health Organization. World Mental Health Report: Transforming Mental Health for All. 2022. Available online: https://www.who.int/publications/i/item/9789240049338 (accessed on 3 March 2025).
Park, S.-H.; Kwak, M.-J. Performance of the Geriatric Depression Scale-15 with Older Adults Aged over 65 Years: An Updated Review 2000–2019. *Clin. Gerontol.* **2020**, *44*, 83–96. [CrossRef]
de Abrantes, G.G.; Souza, G.G.; Cunha, N.M.; da Rocha, H.N.B.; Silva, A.O.; Vasconcelos, S.C. Depressive Symptoms in Older Adults in Basic Health Care. *Rev. Bras. Geriatr. Gerontol.* **2019**, *22*, e190023. [CrossRef]
Uomoto, K.E. Increasing Identification and Follow-up of Older Adult Depression in Primary Care. *J. Prim. Care Community Health* **2023**, *14*, 215013192311527. [CrossRef]

healthcare

MDPI

Review

Fall Risk Assessment and Prevention Strategies in Nursing Homes: A Narrative Review

Takeshi Miura * and Yuka Kanoya

Department of Gerontological Nursing, Nursing Course, School of Medicine, Yokohama City University, Yokohama 236-0004, Japan; ykano@yokohama-cu.ac.jp
* Correspondence: miura.tak.cq@yokohama-cu.ac.jp; Tel.: +81-45-787-2774

Abstract: Abstract: Background/Objectives: Falls in nursing homes significantly affect residents' health and quality of life. Although considerable progress has been made in fall prevention strategies in acute care settings and community environments, research on fall risk assessment methods and prevention strategies in nursing homes remains scarce. Nursing homes provide long-term care for residents with high levels of dependency, presenting unique challenges in managing fall risks. Nevertheless, unlike hospitals, nursing homes face operational constraints, such as limited resources and staffing. These factors necessitate a tailored approach to fall risk management. This study aimed to summarize the current knowledge of fall risk assessment and prevention methods in nursing homes, clarify practical insights for implementation, and identify research gaps based on studies published over the past five years. **Methods:** This narrative review targeted studies published between 2019 and 2024 on fall risk assessment and prevention methods in nursing homes. A literature search was conducted using the PubMed and CINAHL databases, combining keywords such as "Accident Prevention", "Fall Risk Assessment", "Nursing Homes", "Long-Term Care", and "Aged". The inclusion criteria allowed the inclusion of peer-reviewed academic articles on fall risk assessment or prevention interventions in long-term care facilities published in English within the past five years. Studies focusing on community-dwelling older adults, hospitalized older adults, and review articles were excluded. **Results:** This review analyzed 55 studies; among them, 27 studies focused on fall risk assessment and 28 focused on fall prevention. Regarding fall risk assessment, widely used tools, such as the Morse Fall Scale, which is also utilized in medical settings, have been extensively examined. In addition, new predictive methods utilizing electronic health records (EHR) and wearable devices have been introduced. However, the limited number of reports highlights the potential challenges in developing indicators that consider the unique characteristics and feasibility of LTC facilities. Regarding fall prevention, studies have examined indirect approaches, such as environmental modifications, and direct interventions, such as exercise programs. Furthermore, staff education and organizational initiatives are crucial in implementing preventive measures. However, most studies have been conducted in experimental settings, with limited empirical research available to assess the practical applications of these strategies in real-world nursing home environments. **Conclusions:** Fall risk assessments in nursing homes lack practical indicators tailored to the specific characteristics of long-term care facilities. Although various digital technologies have been explored for fall prevention, empirical studies that validate their real-world applicability are lacking.

Keywords: nursing homes; long-term care; falls; risk assessment; fall prevention

1. Introduction

The global population of individuals aged 65 years and older is rapidly increasing compared to other age groups, primarily due to rising life expectancies [1–3]. By 2050, the population of people aged 65 and older is expected to double, while the population of those aged 80 is projected to triple [1]. Older adults, commonly defined as those aged 65 years and older, are at a higher risk of falls and hospitalization compared to other age groups, and the number of older individuals residing in nursing homes is expected to increase in the coming years [4].

Falls are a significant concern in nursing homes, where residents often experience frailty, limited mobility, and multiple chronic conditions [5]. Falls are one of the leading causes of injury and mortality among older adults globally, particularly in institutional care settings such as nursing homes [6]. Research has shown that falls in nursing homes can result in severe physical injuries, a decline in quality of life, and increased healthcare costs [5–8]. Despite developing various fall prevention strategies in hospital and community settings [9–12], there remains a lack of clear and consistent evidence regarding fall prevention in long-term care facilities, particularly those serving highly dependent older adults [13].

The rising incidence of falls in nursing homes imposes a significant burden on residents, healthcare staff, and the overall healthcare system [14]. Nursing homes are designed to provide care for older adults with high dependency levels, presenting unique challenges in managing fall risks [15]. The incidence of falls in long-term care facilities is significantly higher than that in community-dwelling older adults, with an average of 1.7 falls per resident annually, compared to 0.65 falls in private homes. Furthermore, 57.9% of nursing home residents experience at least one fall annually, and 24.2% of these cases result in hospitalization [13,16]. Unlike acute care hospitals, which provide short-term care, nursing homes offer long-term care, making fall prevention an ongoing concern. Practical fall risk assessment in such environments requires a comprehensive understanding of residents' health conditions and the environmental factors contributing to falls. Additionally, fall prevention measures should be feasible and adaptable to the daily operations of nursing homes, where resources and staffing levels may limit the scope of interventions.

This narrative review aims to organize and summarize the current knowledge of fall risk assessment and prevention methods in nursing homes, clarify practical insights for implementation, and identify research gaps based on studies published over the past five years (2019–2024). The findings of this review will serve as a foundation for healthcare professionals, such as physicians and nurses working in elderly care facilities, enabling them to better understand their patients' characteristics and challenges. Furthermore, this review highlights key areas requiring further research to enhance fall prevention strategies in nursing homes.

2. Methods

The literature search period for this review was set from 2019 to 2024, to incorporate the latest research findings in this field. The studies included in this review were selected based on their focus on fall risk assessment methods or fall prevention interventions in nursing homes. A comprehensive literature search was conducted using Medline via PubMed and the CINAHL database to identify relevant studies. The keywords used included combinations of terms such as Accident Prevention, Fall Risk Assessment, Nursing Homes, Long-Term Care, and Aged (Table 1). The researchers developed a draft search strategy for Medline via PubMed in consultation with a medical information specialist. Subsequently, a search strategy for the CINAHL database was constructed based on the search queries used in PubMed (Table 1).

Table 1. Literature search strategy for Medline via PubMed and CINAHL.

	Search Query	Results	Remarks
#1	"Nursing Homes"[MeSH Terms] OR "long term care"[MeSH Terms] OR "Homes for the Aged"[MeSH Terms] OR "nursing home*"[Title/Abstract] OR "long term care"[Title/Abstract] OR "Residential Aged Care Facility"[Title/Abstract] OR "old age home*"[Title/Abstract] OR "Senior Housing"[Title/Abstract]	99,596	nursing homes/long-term car
#2	"Accidental Falls"[MeSH Terms] OR "fall*"[Title/Abstract]	268,521	fall
#3	"Forecasting"[MeSH Terms] OR "Accident Prevention"[MeSH Terms] OR "Risk Assessment"[MeSH Terms] OR "Geriatric Assessment"[MeSH Terms] OR "Digital Technology"[MeSH Terms] OR "Big Data"[MeSH Terms] OR "Data Mining"[MeSH Terms] OR "Datasets as Topic"[MeSH Terms] OR "Data Science"[MeSH Terms] OR "Data Collection"[MeSH Terms] OR "prediction*"[Title/Abstract] OR "prevention*"[Title/Abstract] OR "assessment*"[Title/Abstract] OR "digital technology*"[Title/Abstract] OR "Digital Electronics"[Title/Abstract] OR "Big Data"[Title/Abstract] OR "Data Mining"[Title/Abstract] OR "Text Mining"[Title/Abstract] OR "dataset*"[Title/Abstract] OR "data set*"[Title/Abstract] OR "data science*"[Title/Abstract] OR "data analytic*"[Title/Abstract] OR "Data Collection"[Title/Abstract]	5,585,191	Assessment/Preventic
#4	"Aged"[MeSH Terms] OR "Aged"[Title/Abstract]	4,143,060	Aged
#5	#1 AND #2 AND #3 AND #4	1881	
#6	#5 AND (2019:2024[pdat])	470	2019–2024
Search Strategy: PubMed	(("Nursing Homes"[MeSH Terms] OR "long term care"[MeSH Terms] OR "Homes for the Aged"[MeSH Terms] OR "nursing home*"[Title/Abstract] OR "long term care"[Title/Abstract] OR "Residential Aged Care Facility"[Title/Abstract] OR "old age home*"[Title/Abstract] OR "Senior Housing"[Title/Abstract]) AND ("Accidental Falls"[MeSH Terms] OR "fall*"[Title/Abstract]) AND ("Forecasting"[MeSH Terms] OR "Accident Prevention"[MeSH Terms] OR "Risk Assessment"[MeSH Terms] OR "Geriatric Assessment"[MeSH Terms] OR "Digital Technology"[MeSH Terms] OR "Big Data"[MeSH Terms] OR "Data Mining"[MeSH Terms] OR "Datasets as Topic"[MeSH Terms] OR "Data Science"[MeSH Terms] OR "Data Collection"[MeSH Terms] OR "prediction*"[Title/Abstract] OR "prevention*"[Title/Abstract] OR "assessment*"[Title/Abstract] OR "digital technolog*"[Title/Abstract] OR "Digital Electronics"[Title/Abstract] OR "Big Data"[Title/Abstract] OR "Data Mining"[Title/Abstract] OR "Text Mining"[Title/Abstract] OR "dataset*"[Title/Abstract] OR "data set*"[Title/Abstract] OR "data science*"[Title/Abstract] OR "data analytic*"[Title/Abstract] OR "Data Collection"[Title/Abstract]) AND ("Aged"[MeSH Terms] OR "Aged"[Title/Abstract])) AND (2019:2024[pdat])		
Search Strategy: CINAHL	((MH "Nursing Homes+") OR (MH "Long Term Care") OR TI ("Nursing Home*" OR "Long Term Care" OR "Residential Aged Care Facility" OR "Old Age Home*" OR "Senior Housing") OR AB ("Nursing Home*" OR "Long Term Care" OR "Residential Aged Care Facility" OR "Old Age Home*" OR "Senior Housing")) AND ((MH "Accidental Falls") OR TI fall* OR AB fall*) AND ((MH "Forecasting") OR (MH "Fall Prevention (Iowa NIC)") OR (MH "Risk Assessment") OR (MH "Geriatric Assessment+") OR (MH "Digital Technology+") OR (MH "Data Mining+") OR (MH "Data Science") OR (MH "Data Collection+") OR TI (Prediction* OR Prevention* OR Assessment* OR "Digital Technolog*" OR "Digital Electronics" OR "Big Data" OR "Data Mining" OR "Text Mining" OR Dataset* OR "Data set*" OR "Data Science*" OR "Data Analytic*" OR "Data Collection") OR AB (Prediction* OR Prevention* OR Assessment* OR "Digital Technolog*" OR "Digital Electronics" OR "Big Data" OR "Data Mining" OR "Text Mining" OR Dataset* OR "Data set*" OR "Data Science*" OR "Data Analytic*" OR "Data Collection")) AND ((MH "Aged+") OR TI aged OR AB aged)		

The inclusion criteria for the studies were as follows: (1) peer-reviewed academic articles; (2) published within the past five years; (3) written in English; (4) focusing on long-term care facility settings; and (5) employing observational, interventional, or qualitative research designs. The exclusion criteria were as follows: (1) studies focusing solely on community-dwelling older adults; (2) studies focusing on hospitalized older adults; and (3) systematic or scoping reviews.

A literature search was conducted using the search strategies outlined in Table 1. The initial search yielded 598 articles. The titles and abstracts of these articles were screened to determine their relevance to the scope of this review. As a result, 141, 100, and 55 articles were selected after title, abstract, and full-text review, respectively (Figure 1).

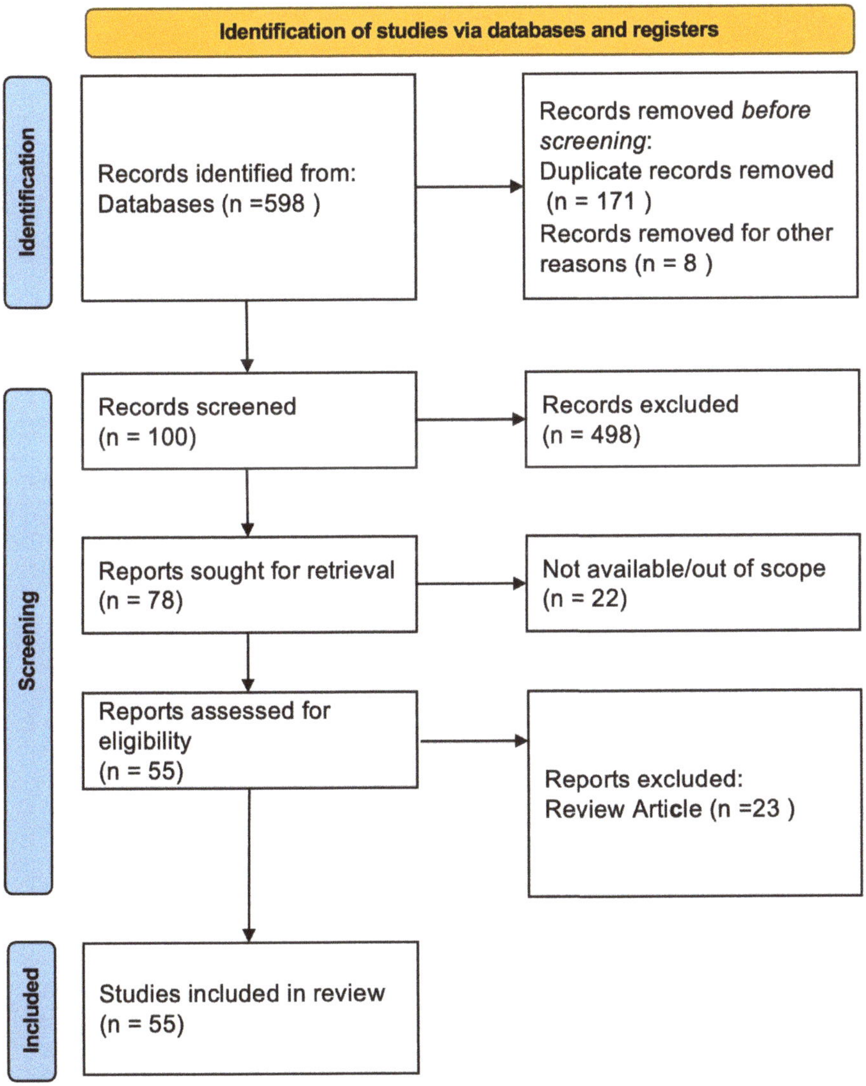

Figure 1. Flow diagram of literature selection process.

The eligible studies included in this review provided detailed descriptions of fall risk assessment tools and prevention strategies specific to nursing homes. The included studies were categorized based on the fall risk assessment and prevention methods on which they focused, organizing similar approaches. By examining these studies, this review clarifies the current trends in fall risk assessment and prevention in nursing homes and highlights their applicability, strengths, and challenges.

3. Results

The 55 reviewed studies were categorized into two main areas: fall risk assessment and fall prevention. Regarding risk assessment, 13 studies focused on risk assessment and indicators [17–29], three on data utilization [30–32], and 11 on the application of digital technologies [33–43]. Regarding fall prevention, six studies addressed environmental adjustments and safety measures [44–49], 17 focused on prevention programs [50–66], and five examined organizational management and staff education [67–71]. The Results section describes the characteristics, indicators, programs, and technologies discussed in these studies.

3.1. Fall Risk Assessment

3.1.1. Risk Assessment and Indicators

The reviewed studies presented various approaches to assessing the fall risk among nursing home residents, ranging from traditional risk assessment tools to advanced assessment methods. Owing to their simplicity, traditional tools continue to be widely used. Among the tools reported were the Morse Fall Scale [18,29], Peninsula Health Falls Risk Assessment Tool [20], Toulouse Saint Louis University Mini Falls Assessment [21], InterRAI Fall Risk Clinical Assessment Protocol [24], Scott Fall Risk Screen [24], Modified Fall Risk Tool [24], Berg Balance Scale [25], Balance Evaluation Systems Test [25], Mini-BESTest [25], Brief-BESTest [25], STOP-FALLING checklist [26], and Injury Risk in Nursing Homes tool [28]. These tools assess mobility restriction, cognitive impairment, and medication use.

Additionally, studies have explored methods to assess fall risks based on the gait conditions of residents [17,27], using electronic health records to identify at-risk individuals [19]. Research evaluating gait patterns has emphasized their value in assessing fall risks, whereas electronic health record (EHR)-based methods have highlighted the potential to monitor and assess the risk dynamically by integrating data.

These findings highlight the importance of various approaches, ranging from foundational tools to cutting-edge technologies. Although traditional tools remain indispensable for baseline assessments, technologies such as gait analysis and assessment methods using EHRs are being explored to address the complex and ever-changing health conditions of nursing home residents. These findings can contribute to fall risk assessments tailored to the characteristics of nursing home residents and to the selection of effective intervention strategies based on these assessments.

3.1.2. Data Utilization

The use of EHRs and large-scale data for fall risk assessment has garnered increased attention. Routinely collected EHRs can serve as dynamic and comprehensive tools for risk assessment and management in nursing homes. The reviewed studies have investigated fall risk assessment models using routinely collected data and administrative datasets [30–32].

A study using EHR data developed and internally validated a dynamic fall risk assessment and monitoring tool in aged care settings, focusing on methods of dynamically evaluating the constructed models [30]. Another study utilized the Minimum Data Set (MDS) from nursing homes to develop a fall risk assessment model. This model incorporated factors such as medication data, the use of walking aids, and physical function to assess the fall risk within 90 days [31]. Furthermore, another study leveraging healthcare system data measured fall-related injuries and developed measurement models [32].

Despite these advancements, some challenges must still be overcome when implementing EHR-based risk assessment models. Many nursing homes lack the infrastructure to utilize these systems fully, and staff training is critical to ensure accurate data entry and interpretation. Moreover, addressing privacy and data security concerns is essential to building trust and ensuring the ethical use of resident information. The reviewed studies emphasized the value of routinely collected EHR data in developing dynamic, accurate, and scalable fall risk assessment tools. Nursing homes can effectively enhance their capacity to assess and manage fall risks by utilizing existing datasets and advanced measurement models. However, the limited number of studies and the remaining challenges indicate that further efforts are needed to develop practical methods that nursing professionals can readily adopt.

3.1.3. Use of Digital Devices

The reviewed studies highlighted various digital devices used in fall risk assessment and prevention in nursing homes, demonstrating their potential to complement traditional methods through real-time monitoring and analytical capabilities, ultimately leading to more effective assessments by nursing staff. Wearable devices have been a common focus, with reports on their ability to evaluate mobility and balance. For instance, a spatiotemporal gait analysis validated the G-STRIDE inertial sensor for the assessment of fall risks [36]. Similarly, the Smart Belt demonstrated the potential to mitigate the impact of falls by monitoring movement patterns and deploying airbags to reduce hip injuries during falls [37]. Smartphone-based gait analysis systems such as the mVEGAS have also been validated in identifying mobility impairments in various settings [39]. Additionally, the MoTFall project showcased the integration of applications and sensors to address fall risks [40]. In Bangkok, a robotics-based fall prevention program improved knowledge, promoted exercise, and enhanced balance among older adults, thereby reducing fall incidents [43]. Furthermore, cost-effective activity trackers helped to track daily activities and fall risk indicators in resource-limited environments [41].

These studies illustrate the expanding role of wearable devices, sensors, and robotics in fall risk assessment and prevention in nursing homes. These devices can facilitate efficient nursing assessments, even with constrained resources in resident-centered care settings, where limited staff must manage many residents.

3.2. Fall Prevention Methods

3.2.1. Environmental Adjustments and Safety

The reviewed studies highlighted a range of environmental adjustments and safety measures to reduce fall risks in nursing homes, emphasizing their impacts and practical implementation challenges. A study in Shanghai highlighted environmental hazards such as poor lighting and uneven floors as significant contributors to falls, advocating for systematic facility-wide improvements [47]. Upgraded lighting, including motion-sensitive systems, demonstrated significant fall rate reductions and boosted residents' confidence in nighttime navigation [45]. Wearable safety devices such as hip airbags effectively reduce the severity of fall-related injuries in long-term care facilities [46,49]. However, varying perceptions regarding the use of hip protectors have also been revealed [48]. Specialized equipment such as lifting cushions has proven valuable in reducing complications and caregiver strain by assisting fallen residents [44]. These studies underscore the importance of environmental adjustments and targeted safety measures as foundational strategies for fall prevention in nursing homes.

3.2.2. Fall Prevention Programs

In addition to programs with proven effectiveness, such as the Otago Exercise Program [65], new interventional programs, such as the Staying UpRight [58] and SUNBEAM programs [61], have shown the potential to improve residents' stability. Tai Chi has also been suggested to reduce the fear of movement [55]. Furthermore, the effectiveness of volunteer-supported walking programs [57], leisure activities [62], and music-based programs [66] has been validated. Multifactorial interventions that combine various approaches have recently gained attention [54,64]. These exercise-integrated programs highlight the importance of preventive measures in communities, healthcare settings, and older adult care facilities.

3.2.3. Organizational Management and Staff Education

The reviewed studies emphasized the importance of organizational management and staff education in fall prevention strategies within long-term care facilities, highlighting the roles of staff training, interdisciplinary collaboration, and leadership support. Frequent and concise training sessions ("brief but often") were found effective in enhancing staff skills and maintaining engagement, particularly in the use of risk assessment tools and safe transfer techniques [67]. A cross-sectional study highlighted the variability in staff confidence levels, showing the need for targeted training to address gaps in the understanding of environmental hazards and monitoring technologies [68]. These measures have been linked to a reduction in fall incidents.

Interdisciplinary approaches such as the Training In Policy Studies program have demonstrated the benefits of personalized fall prevention strategies developed collaboratively by nurses, physiotherapists, and other professionals [69]. Integrating nurse practitioners into care facilities enhanced fall risk management, offering cost savings and improved resident outcomes through medication reviews and staff mentorship [70]. Ethical and operational challenges, such as staff acceptance of new technologies and privacy concerns, were also identified. Leadership commitment was critical in ensuring the smooth and ethical implementation of safety practices [71].

Overall, these studies highlight that effective fall prevention requires strong leadership, continuous education, and teamwork, as well as addressing operational and ethical challenges.

4. Discussion

4.1. Fall Risk Assessment

Fall risk assessment in nursing homes remains a critical priority because of its significant implications for residents' health and quality of life. This review points out that research on fall risk assessment tools in nursing homes is limited compared to studies conducted in other settings, highlighting the need to address this gap. Traditional tools such as the Morse Fall Scale (MFS) and Peninsular Health Falls Risk Assessment Tool (PH-FRAT) continue to be widely utilized because of their simplicity and cost-effectiveness [18,20]. These tools evaluate essential factors, including mobility limitations, cognitive impairments, and medication use, providing a foundational framework for the identification of fall risks. However, their static nature and inability to capture daily fluctuations in the health conditions of residents, such as acute illnesses, medication side effects, and functional changes, pose significant limitations [72]. The reviewed studies also suggested that these tools may underperform in populations with specific needs, such as residents with cognitive impairments, indicating the need for tailored refinements [73]. Various fall risk assessment tools have been developed and validated for hospitalized patients and community-dwelling older adults; however, a review of studies from the past five years focusing on nursing homes revealed that reports specific to these settings still need to be made available. Further research is anticipated to support the development of more effective assessment tools tailored to the unique needs of nursing home residents [9,74–76].

In contrast to the extensive research in acute care hospitals, which often utilize large-scale healthcare databases to develop advanced assessment indicators, progress in nursing homes remains comparatively lacking [77–79]. This disparity is attributed to the need for standardized observational indicators specific to nursing homes and the absence of comprehensive databases. Bridging this gap requires the development of unified data-collection frameworks and investment in large-scale datasets tailored to nursing home populations. However, the implementation of such systems is hindered by challenges such as insufficient technological infrastructure in nursing homes, staff training needs, and concerns about data privacy and security [80].

Wearable devices and environmental sensors provide additional opportunities to enhance fall risk assessments. Devices such as the G-STRIDE inertial sensor, the Smart Belt, and smartphone-based systems enable the continuous monitoring of gait patterns, mobility, and physiological parameters [36,37]. These technologies complement EHR systems by adding real-time data to improve the assessment accuracy. However, their widespread adoption faces financial constraints, resident resistance, and maintenance challenges.

4.1.1. Fall Prevention Methods

Fall prevention in nursing homes requires flexible strategies that integrate environmental, physical, and organizational approaches to address the diverse cognitive functions and daily life activities of residents.

Environmental modifications form the foundation of fall prevention [81]. Simple interventions can reduce fall rates by eliminating tripping hazards, installing handrails, and introducing motion-sensitive lighting [82]. Advanced measures, including non-slip flooring, automated bed sensors, and wearable devices such as hip airbags, can further mitigate the severity of fall-related injuries. Exercise programs also play a pivotal role in fall prevention [83,84]. Interventions such as the Otago Exercise Program [65] and SUNBEAM [61] have significantly improved the physical stability of residents and reduced the fall rates. Additionally, Tai Chi, which has been validated in numerous studies, effectively enhances balance, reduces fear of movement, and improves cognitive function [55]. This dual benefit is particularly advantageous for residents with mild cognitive impairment as it supports physical and mental health. Combining these programs with complementary strategies such as medication reviews and staff education further amplifies their effectiveness. However, individualized program designs are indispensable in addressing the diversity of physical and cognitive conditions among residents. Organizational strategies and staff education are critical in effectively implementing fall prevention measures [67–71,85]. Frequent and concise training sessions help to maintain staff knowledge and skills [67]. The implementation of such programs requires substantial resources. Collaboration with external organizations and community health initiatives can play a crucial role in overcoming these constraints. For example, involving physiotherapy students or volunteers can help to alleviate staff's workloads while maintaining program quality [57]. In conclusion, fall prevention in nursing homes requires a comprehensive approach that integrates environmental adjustments, exercise programs, cognitive interventions, and organizational strategies. Although challenges related to resource limitations and resident acceptance persist, innovative and evidence-based solutions hold great potential in improving residents' safety and quality of life. Future research should focus on developing scalable, sustainable, and individualized interventions to address these barriers effectively.

4.1.2. Future Directions in Research

Research on fall risk assessment and prevention in care facilities faces numerous challenges but holds significant potential to improve safety and care quality. Several key directions for future research have been identified. First, it is essential to standardize fall risk assessment. The development of simple and universally applicable tools that can be seamlessly integrated into daily workflows is expected to ensure consistency in evaluations across facilities, enhance the assessment accuracy, and reduce staff workloads [86]. Data integration and infrastructure development are critical issues. Establishing centralized systems to aggregate and share data from care facilities would enable the efficient tracking of fall incidents and the practical analysis of interventional outcomes. Achieving this requires investments in data sharing infrastructure and the establishment of ethical governance frameworks. Furthermore, translating research findings into practical applications is vital. Although the effectiveness of many fall prevention strategies, such as exercise programs, medication reviews, and environmental modifications, has been demonstrated in controlled settings, adapting these strategies to real-world constraints necessitates the development of sustainable models. Moreover, a comprehensive approach that addresses the complex needs of the residents is crucial. The integration of the physical, cognitive, emotional, and social dimensions into prevention strategies can provide tailored care. Interdisciplinary collaboration among healthcare professionals is the key to delivering holistic care that meets the individual needs of residents [87]. Finally, technological innovation plays an important role. Wearable devices, EHRs, and environmental sensors offer opportunities for continuous monitoring and proactive interventions. However, challenges, such as costs, user resistance, and inadequate digital infrastructure, must be addressed. Collaboration between technology developers and care providers is essential in establishing practical and actionable interventional methods suitable for real-world implementation. Addressing these challenges can enhance the safety and efficacy of fall prevention in care facilities while aligning with advancements in other healthcare fields. Future research should prioritize the development of practical evidence-based assessment and prevention strategies that align with these directions to deliver high-quality care in care settings.

5. Conclusions

This review highlights the current state and challenges in fall risk assessment and prevention in nursing homes. Research on fall risk assessment remains insufficient in terms of considering the specific setting of this field while ensuring its feasibility. Moreover, the absence of standardized indicators and large-scale databases for verification poses a significant barrier to progress in this area. Future research should prioritize the development of fall risk assessment indicators tailored to the unique characteristics of long-term care facilities. These indicators should be designed to be practical and easy to understand, not only for nursing professionals but also for caregivers and a diverse range of healthcare and long-term care staff.

Existing evidence demonstrates the effectiveness of exercise interventions. However, considering the ongoing aging of the population and the increasing shortage of healthcare and caregiving staff, conventional approaches alone may not be sufficient as sustainable fall prevention strategies. Therefore, establishing more effective and efficient methods that incorporate digital technology is essential. Real-time monitoring using wearable devices and environmental sensors has the potential to facilitate the early detection of fall risks and enable individualized interventions, contributing to the optimal use of limited resources.

On the other hand, although the implementation of digital technologies is progressing to some extent, most existing studies have been conducted in experimental settings, raising concerns about the safety and effectiveness of these technologies in real-world applications. Future research should focus on promoting practical studies that evaluate these technologies in actual nursing home environments and incorporate the perspectives of both caregivers and residents. Furthermore, successful implementation requires improvements in technological infrastructure, enhanced staff training programs, and the establishment of frameworks that address data privacy and ethical considerations.

The findings of this review suggest that the key future directions for fall risk assessment and prevention in nursing homes include the development of evidence-based assessment tools, establishment of innovative approaches leveraging digital technologies, and promotion of practical studies to ensure their applicability in real-world settings. These efforts are expected to enhance the effectiveness of fall prevention measures and improve the safety and quality of life of nursing home residents.

Limitation

This study had several limitations. Since the primary aim of this review was to present recent evidence to readers, this restricted the scope of the literature databases and the time frame considered. Consequently, relevant studies might have been overlooked. Additionally, it should be noted that evidence has yet to be integrated. To ensure the quality of this narrative review, we adhered to the SANRA scale [88] and tried to provide unbiased and reliable information.

Author Contributions: T.M. conceptualized the review and drafted the manuscript. T.M. and Y.K. contributed to the review of the relevant literature and manuscript editing. All authors have read and agreed to the published version of the manuscript.

Funding: This research received no external funding.

Institutional Review Board Statement: Not applicable. Ethical approval was not required because this review did not involve human or animal subjects.

Informed Consent Statement: Not applicable. No human participants were involved in this review.

Conflicts of Interest: The authors declare no conflicts of interest related to this research.

eferences

World Health Organization. Ageing and Health. Available online: https://www.who.int/news-room/fact-sheets/detail/ageing-and-health (accessed on 2 December 2024).
Tohit, N.F.M.; Haque, M. The new frontier of ageing: Innovations and insights in gerontology. *Adv. Hum. Biol.* **2024**, *14*, 261–268. [CrossRef]
Roberts, L.W. Preparing for the Needs of Our Aging Population. *Acad. Med.* **2024**, *99*, 123–125. [CrossRef] [PubMed]
World Health Organization. Falls. Available online: https://www.who.int/news-room/fact-sheets/detail/falls (accessed on 2 December 2024).
Xu, D.; Wang, Y.; Zhu, S.; Zhao, M.; Wang, K. Relationship between fear of falling and quality of life in nursing home residents: The role of activity restriction. *Geriatr. Nurs.* **2024**, *57*, 45–50. [CrossRef] [PubMed]
Shao, L.; Shi, Y.; Xie, X.Y.; Wang, Z.; Wang, Z.A.; Zhang, J.E. Incidence and Risk Factors of Falls Among Older People in Nursing Homes: Systematic Review and Meta-Analysis. *J. Am. Med. Dir. Assoc.* **2023**, *24*, 1708–1717. [CrossRef]
. Saljuqi, A.T.; Anand, T.; Joseph, B. Reassessing the economic burden of geriatric falls: A call for preventive action. *Trauma. Surg. Acute Care Open* **2024**, *9*, e001591. [CrossRef]
. Sterke, C.S.; Panneman, M.J.; Erasmus, V.; Polinder, S.; van Beeck, E.F. Increased care demand and medical costs after falls in nursing homes: A Delphi study. *J. Clin. Nurs.* **2018**, *27*, 2896–2903. [CrossRef]
. Colón-Emeric, C.S.; McDermott, C.L.; Lee, D.S.; Berry, S.D. Risk Assessment and Prevention of Falls in Older Community-Dwelling Adults: A Review. *JAMA* **2024**, *331*, 1397–1406. [CrossRef]
0. US Preventive Services Task Force; Grossman, D.C.; Curry, S.J.; Owens, D.K.; Barry, M.J.; Caughey, A.B.; Davidson, K.W.; Doubeni, C.A.; Epling, J.W., Jr.; Kemper, A.R.; et al. Interventions to Prevent Falls in Community-Dwelling Older Adults: US Preventive Services Task Force Recommendation Statement. *JAMA* **2018**, *319*, 1696–1704. [CrossRef]

11. Dykes, P.C.; Curtin-Bowen, M.; Lipsitz, S.; Franz, C.; Adelman, J.; Adkison, L.; Bogaisky, M.; Carroll, D.; Carter, E.; Herlihy, et al. Cost of Inpatient Falls and Cost-Benefit Analysis of Implementation of an Evidence-Based Fall Prevention Program. *JAM Health Forum* **2023**, *4*, e225125. [CrossRef]
12. Morris, M.E.; Webster, K.; Jones, C.; Hill, A.M.; Haines, T.; McPhail, S.; Kiegaldie, D.; Slade, S.; Jazayeri, D.; Heng, H.; et Interventions to reduce falls in hospitals: A systematic review and meta-analysis. *Age Ageing* **2022**, *51*, afac077. [CrossRef]
13. Parekh, A.; Hill, K.D.; Guerbaai, R.A. Exploring Post-Fall Management Interventions in Long-Term Care Facilities and Hospit for Older Adults: A Scoping Rreview. *J. Clin. Nurs.* **2024**, *34*, 408–421. [CrossRef] [PubMed]
14. Kimura, M.; Ruller, S.; Frank, C.; Bell, A.; Jacobson, M.; Pardo, J.P.; Ramsey, T.; Sobala, M.; Fung, C.; Kobewka, D. Inciden Morbidity and Mortality From Falls in Skilled Nursing Facilities: A Systematic Review and Meta-Analysis. *J. Am. Med. Dir. Ass* **2023**, *24*, 1690–1699.e6. [CrossRef] [PubMed]
15. Salari, N.; Darvishi, N.; Ahmadipanah, M.; Shohaimi, S.; Mohammadi, M. Global prevalence of falls in the older adults: comprehensive systematic review and meta-analysis. *J. Orthop. Surg. Res.* **2022**, *17*, 334. [CrossRef] [PubMed]
16. Cameron, I.D.; Dyer, S.M.; Panagoda, C.E.; Murray, G.R.; Hill, K.D.; Cumming, R.G.; Kerse, N. Interventions for preventing fa in older people in care facilities and hospitals. *Cochrane Database Syst. Rev.* **2018**, *9*, CD005465. [CrossRef]
17. Jia, S.; Si, Y.; Guo, C.; Wang, P.; Li, S.; Wang, J.; Wang, X. The prediction model of fall risk for the elderly based on gait analys *BMC Public Health* **2024**, *24*, 2206. [CrossRef]
18. Liu, J.; Luo, Y.; Chai, X.; Zeng, S.; Liu, Y.; Zhao, L. Rasch analysis of Morse Fall Scale among the older adults with cogniti impairment in nursing homes. *Geriatr. Nurs.* **2024**, *56*, 94–99. [CrossRef]
19. Berry, S.D.; Hecker, E.J.; McConnell, E.S.; Xue, T.M.; Tsai, T.; Zullo, A.R.; Colón-Emeric, C.; Nursing Home, P. Revention of Inju in DEmentia (NH PRIDE): A pilot study of a remote injury prevention service for NH residents. *J. Am. Geriatr. Soc.* **2023**, *7* 3267–3277. [CrossRef]
20. Wabe, N.; Siette, J.; Seaman, K.L.; Nguyen, A.D.; Raban, M.Z.; Close, J.C.T.; Lord, S.R.; Westbrook, J.I. The use and predicti performance of the Peninsula Health Falls Risk Assessment Tool (PH-FRAT) in 25 residential aged care facilities: A retrospecti cohort study using routinely collected data. *BMC Geriatr.* **2022**, *22*, 271. [CrossRef]
21. Locquet, M.; Bonnard, F.; Beaudart, C.; Coendo, C.; Gillain, S.; Reginster, J.Y.; Bruyère, O. An Assessment of the Toulouse Sai Louis University Mini Falls Assessment Tool to Predict Incident Falls among Older Adults Residing in Nursing Homes: 6-Month Prospective Study. *J. Nutr. Health Aging* **2021**, *25*, 933–937. [CrossRef]
22. Michalcova, J.; Vasut, K.; Airaksinen, M.; Bielakova, K. Inclusion of medication-related fall risk in fall risk assessment tool i geriatric care units. *BMC Geriatr.* **2020**, *20*, 454. [CrossRef]
23. Charles, A.; Buckinx, F.; Locquet, M.; Reginster, J.Y.; Petermans, J.; Gruslin, B.; Bruyère, O. Prediction of Adverse Outcomes i Nursing Home Residents According to Intrinsic Capacity Proposed by the World Health Organization. *J. Gerontol. A Biol. Sc Med. Sci.* **2020**, *75*, 1594–1599. [CrossRef] [PubMed]
24. Norman, K.J.; Hirdes, J.P. Evaluation of the Predictive Accuracy of the interRAI Falls Clinical Assessment Protocol, Scott Fall Ris Screen, and a Supplementary Falls Risk Assessment Tool Used in Residential Long-Term Care: A Retrospective Cohort Stud *Can. J. Aging* **2020**, *39*, 521–532. [CrossRef] [PubMed]
25. Viveiro, L.A.P.; Gomes, G.C.V.; Bacha, J.M.R.; Carvas Junior, N.; Kallas, M.E.; Reis, M.; Jacob Filho, W.; Pompeu, J.E. Reliability Validity, and Ability to Identity Fall Status of the Berg Balance Scale, Balance Evaluation Systems Test (BESTest), Mini-BESTes and Brief-BESTest in Older Adults Who Live in Nursing Homes. *J. Geriatr. Phys. Ther.* **2019**, *42*, E45–E54. [CrossRef] [PubMed]
26. Wongrakpanich, S.; Danji, K.; Lipsitz, L.; Berry, S. STOP-FALLING: A Simple Checklist Tool for Fall Prevention in a Nursing Facility. *J. Am. Med. Dir. Assoc.* **2019**, *20*, 916–918. [CrossRef]
27. Fien, S.; Henwood, T.; Climstein, M.; Rathbone, E.; Keogh, J.W.L. Gait Speed Characteristics and Their Spatiotemporal Determi nants in Nursing Home Residents: A Cross-Sectional Study. *J. Geriatr. Phys. Ther.* **2019**, *42*, E148–E154. [CrossRef]
28. Duprey, M.S.; Zullo, A.R.; Gouskova, N.A.; Lee, Y.; Capuano, A.; Kiel, D.P.; Daiello, L.A.; Kim, D.H.; Berry, S.D. Development and validation of the fall-related injury risk in nursing homes (INJURE-NH) prediction tool. *J. Am. Geriatr. Soc.* **2023**, *71*, 1851–1860 [CrossRef]
29. Zeleníková, R.; Jarošová, D. The predictive validity of the Morse Fall Scale in hospitalized patients in the Czech Republic *Pielęgniarstwo XXI Wieku. Nurs. 21st Century* **2024**, *23*, 86–91. [CrossRef]
30. Wabe, N.; Meulenbroeks, I.; Huang, G.; Silva, S.M.; Gray, L.C.; Close, J.C.T.; Lord, S.; Westbrook, J.I. Development and internal validation of a dynamic fall risk prediction and monitoring tool in aged care using routinely collected electronic health data: A landmarking approach. *J. Am. Med. Inform. Assoc.* **2024**, *31*, 1113–1125. [CrossRef]
31. Boyce, R.D.; Kravchenko, O.V.; Perera, S.; Karp, J.F.; Kane-Gill, S.L.; Reynolds, C.F.; Albert, S.M.; Handler, S.M. Falls prediction using the nursing home minimum dataset. *J. Am. Med. Inform. Assoc.* **2022**, *29*, 1497–1507. [CrossRef]
32. Min, L.; Tinetti, M.; Langa, K.M.; Ha, J.; Alexander, N.; Hoffman, G.J. Measurement of Fall Injury With Health Care System Data and Assessment of Inclusiveness and Validity of Measurement Models. *JAMA Netw. Open* **2019**, *2*, e199679. [CrossRef]

Jain, S.; Burke, C. Falls Prevention Using AI and Remote Surveillance in Nursing Homes. *J. Am. Med. Dir. Assoc.* **2024**, *25*, 105082. [CrossRef] [PubMed]

Can, B.; Tufan, A.; Karadağ, Ş.; DurmuŞ, N.Ş.; Topçu, M.; Aysevinç, B.; Düzel, S.Ç.; Dağcıoğlu, S.; Afşar Fak, N.; Tazegül, G.; et al. The effectiveness of a fall detection device in older nursing home residents: A pilot study. *Psychogeriatrics* **2024**, *24*, 822–829. [CrossRef] [PubMed]

Blasco-García, J.D.; García-López, G.; Jiménez-Muñoz, M.; López-Riquelme, J.A.; Feliu-Batlle, J.J.; Pavón-Pulido, N.; Herrero, M.T. A Computer Vision-Based System to Help Health Professionals to Apply Tests for Fall Risk Assessment. *Sensors* **2024**, *24*, 2015. [CrossRef] [PubMed]

Álvarez, M.N.; Rodríguez-Sánchez, C.; Huertas-Hoyas, E.; García-Villamil-Neira, G.; Espinoza-Cerda, M.T.; Pérez-Delgado, L.; Reina-Robles, E.; Martin, I.B.; Del-Ama, A.J.; Ruiz-Ruiz, L.; et al. Predictors of fall risk in older adults using the G-STRIDE inertial sensor: An observational multicenter case-control study. *BMC Geriatr.* **2023**, *23*, 737. [CrossRef]

Tarbert, R.J.; Singhatat, W. Real World Evidence of Wearable Smartbelt for Mitigation of Fall Impact in Older Adult Care. *IEEE J. Transl. Eng. Health Med.* **2023**, *11*, 247–251. [CrossRef]

Dierick, F.; Stoffel, P.L.; Schütz, G.; Buisseret, F. High Specificity of Single Inertial Sensor-Supplemented Timed Up and Go Test for Assessing Fall Risk in Elderly Nursing Home Residents. *Sensors* **2022**, *22*, 2339. [CrossRef]

Ippisch, R.; Jelusic, A.; Bertram, J.; Schniepp, R.; Wuehr, M. mVEGAS—Mobile smartphone-based spatiotemporal gait analysis in healthy and ataxic gait disorders. *Gait Posture* **2022**, *97*, 80–85. [CrossRef]

Möller, U.O.; Fänge, A.M.; Hansson, E.E. Modern technology against falls—A description of the MoTFall project. *Health Inform. J.* **2021**, *27*, 14604582211011514. [CrossRef]

Unger, E.W.; Histing, T.; Rollmann, M.F.; Orth, M.; Herath, E.; Menger, M.; Herath, S.C.; Grimm, B.; Pohlemann, T.; Braun, B.J. Development of a dynamic fall risk profile in elderly nursing home residents: A free field gait analysis based study. *Arch. Gerontol. Geriatr.* **2021**, *93*, 104294. [CrossRef]

Miranda-Duro, M.D.C.; Nieto-Riveiro, L.; Concheiro-Moscoso, P.; Groba, B.; Pousada, T.; Canosa, N.; Pereira, J. Analysis of Older Adults in Spanish Care Facilities, Risk of Falling and Daily Activity Using Xiaomi Mi Band 2. *Sensors* **2021**, *21*, 3341. [CrossRef]

Maneeprom, N.; Taneepanichskul, S.; Panza, A.; Suputtitada, A. Effectiveness of robotics fall prevention program among elderly in senior housings, Bangkok, Thailand: A quasi-experimental study. *Clin. Interv. Aging* **2019**, *14*, 335–346. [CrossRef] [PubMed]

Houghton, R.; Cowdell, F.; Fry, D.; Dyson, J. Implementation and Impact of a Lifting Cushion for Care Home Residents Who Have Fallen. *Int. J. Older People Nurs.* **2024**, *19*, e12664. [CrossRef] [PubMed]

Grant, L.K.; St Hilaire, M.A.; Heller, J.P.; Heller, R.A.; Lockley, S.W.; Rahman, S.A. Impact of Upgraded Lighting on Falls in Care Home Residents. *J. Am. Med. Dir. Assoc.* **2022**, *23*, 1698–1704.e2. [CrossRef] [PubMed]

Nemeth, B.; van der Kaaij, M.; Nelissen, R.; van Wijnen, J.K.; Drost, K.; Blauw, G.J. Prevention of hip fractures in older adults residing in long-term care facilities with a hip airbag: A retrospective pilot study. *BMC Geriatr.* **2022**, *22*, 547. [CrossRef]

Jiang, Y.; Xia, Q.; Zhou, P.; Jiang, S.; Diwan, V.K.; Xu, B. Environmental hazards increase the fall risk among residents of long-term care facilities: A prospective study in Shanghai, China. *Age Ageing* **2021**, *50*, 875–881. [CrossRef]

3. Hall, A.; Boulton, E.; Stanmore, E. Older adults' perceptions of wearable technology hip protectors: Implications for further research and development strategies. *Disabil. Rehabil. Assist. Technol.* **2019**, *14*, 663–668. [CrossRef]

Korall, A.M.B.; Feldman, F.; Yang, Y.; Cameron, I.D.; Leung, P.M.; Sims-Gould, J.; Robinovitch, S.N. Effectiveness of Hip Protectors to Reduce Risk for Hip Fracture from Falls in Long-Term Care. *J. Am. Med. Dir. Assoc.* **2019**, *20*, 1397–1403.e1. [CrossRef]

Taylor, L.M.; Parsons, J.; Moyes, S.A.; Binns, E.; Cavadino, A.; Taylor, D.; Lord, S.; Del Din, S.; Klenk, J.; Rochester, L.; et al. Effects of an Exercise Program to Reduce Falls in Older People Living in Long-Term Care: A Randomized Controlled Trial. *J. Am. Med. Dir. Assoc.* **2024**, *25*, 201–208.e6. [CrossRef]

1. Suen, J.; Dawson, R.; Kneale, D.; Kwok, W.; Sherrington, C.; Sutcliffe, K.; Cameron, I.D.; Dyer, S.M. Qualitative Comparative Analysis of exercise interventions for fall prevention in residential aged care facilities. *BMC Geriatr.* **2024**, *24*, 728. [CrossRef]

2. Kp, N.; D, A.; Nawed, A.; Nuhmani, S.; Khan, M.; Alghadir, A.H. Comparison of effects of Otago exercise program vs gaze stability exercise on balance and fear of fall in older adults: A randomized trial. *Medicine* **2024**, *103*, e38345. [CrossRef]

3. Baixinho, C.L.; Madeira, C.; Alves, S.; Henriques, M.A.; Dixe, M.D.A. Falls and Preventive Practices among Institutionalized Older People. *Int. J. Environ. Res. Public. Health* **2022**, *19*, 7577. [CrossRef] [PubMed]

4. Logan, P.A.; Horne, J.C.; Gladman, J.R.F.; Gordon, A.L.; Sach, T.; Clark, A.; Robinson, K.; Armstrong, S.; Stirling, S.; Leighton, P.; et al. Multifactorial falls prevention programme compared with usual care in UK care homes for older people: Multicentre cluster randomised controlled trial with economic evaluation. *BMJ* **2021**, *375*, e066991. [CrossRef] [PubMed]

5. Birimoglu Okuyan, C.; Deveci, E. The effectiveness of Tai Chi Chuan on fear of movement, prevention of falls, physical activity, and cognitive status in older adults with mild cognitive impairment: A randomized controlled trial. *Perspect. Psychiatr. Care* **2021**, *57*, 1273–1281, Erratum in *Perspect. Psychiatr. Care* **2022**, *58*, 3118. [CrossRef]

6. Park, B.M. Development and Effect of a Fall Prevention Program Based on King's Theory of Goal Attainment in Long-Term Care Hospitals: An Experimental Study. *Healthcare* **2021**, *9*, 715. [CrossRef]

57. Grede, N.; Trampisch, U.; Weissbach, S.; Heinzel-Gutenbrunner, M.; Freiberger, E.; Sönnichsen, A.; Donner-Banzhoff, N. volunteer-supported walking programme to improve physical function in older people with restricted mobility (the POW Study): A randomised controlled trial. *BMC Geriatr.* **2024**, *24*, 60. [CrossRef]
58. Taylor, L.; Parsons, J.; Taylor, D.; Binns, E.; Lord, S.; Edlin, R.; Rochester, L.; Del Din, S.; Klenk, J.; Buckley, C.; et al. Evaluati the effects of an exercise program (Staying UpRight) for older adults in long-term care on rates of falls: Study protocol fo randomised controlled trial. *Trials* **2020**, *21*, 46. [CrossRef]
59. Toots, A.; Wiklund, R.; Littbrand, H.; Nordin, E.; Nordström, P.; Lundin-Olsson, L.; Gustafson, Y.; Rosendahl, E. The Effects Exercise on Falls in Older People With Dementia Living in Nursing Homes: A Randomized Controlled Trial. *J. Am. Med. L Assoc.* **2019**, *20*, 835–842.e1. [CrossRef]
60. Arrieta, H.; Rezola-Pardo, C.; Gil, S.M.; Virgala, J.; Iturburu, M.; Antón, I.; González-Templado, V.; Irazusta, J.; Rodriguez-Larra A. Effects of Multicomponent Exercise on Frailty in Long-Term Nursing Homes: A Randomized Controlled Trial. *J. Am. Geri Soc.* **2019**, *67*, 1145–1151. [CrossRef]
61. Hewitt, J.; Saing, S.; Goodall, S.; Henwood, T.; Clemson, L.; Refshauge, K. An economic evaluation of the SUNBEAM programm A falls-prevention randomized controlled trial in residential aged care. *Clin. Rehabil.* **2019**, *33*, 524–534. [CrossRef]
62. Huang, G.; Wabe, N.; Raban, M.Z.; Silva, S.S.M.; Seaman, K.; Nguyen, A.D.; Meulenbroeks, I.; Westbrook, J.I. The relationsh between participation in leisure activities and incidence of falls in residential aged care. *PLoS ONE* **2024**, *19*, e0302678. [CrossRe
63. Azkia, Z.; Setiyani, R.; Kusumawardani, L.H. Balance strategy exercise versus lower limb-ROM exercise for reducing the risk falls among older people. *Nurs. Med. J. Nurs.* **2021**, *11*, 114–123. [CrossRef]
64. Courel-Ibáñez, J.; Buendía-Romero, Á.; Pallarés, J.G.; García-Conesa, S.; Martínez-Cava, A.; Izquierdo, M. Impact of Tailore Multicomponent Exercise for Preventing Weakness and Falls on Nursing Home Residents' Functional Capacity. *J. Am. Med. D Assoc.* **2022**, *23*, 98–104.e3. [CrossRef] [PubMed]
65. Zou, Z.; Chen, Z.; Ni, Z.; Hou, Y.; Zhang, Q. The effect of group-based Otago exercise program on fear of falling and physic function among older adults living in nursing homes: A pilot trial. *Geriatr. Nurs.* **2022**, *43*, 288–292. [CrossRef] [PubMed]
66. Odufuwa-Pelote, A.; Johnson, K.; Jones, S.; Carter, H. Effects of music therapy in reducing falls among patients with dementia i a long-term facility: A cohort study. *Nurs. Resid. Care* **2024**, *26*, 1–8. [CrossRef]
67. Albasha, N.; Curtin, C.; McCullagh, R.; Cornally, N.; Timmons, S. Staff perspectives on fall prevention activities in long-term ca facilities for older residents: "Brief but often" staff education is key. *PLoS ONE* **2024**, *19*, e0310139. [CrossRef]
68. Albasha, N.; McCullagh, R.; Cornally, N.; Timmons, S. Staff knowledge, attitudes and confidence levels for fall preventions i older person long-term care facilities: A cross-sectional study. *BMC Geriatr.* **2023**, *23*, 595. [CrossRef]
69. Tzeng, H.M.; Jansen, L.S.; Okpalauwaekwe, U.; Khasnabish, S.; Andreas, B.; Dykes, P.C. Adopting the Fall Tailoring Intervention for Patient Safety (TIPS) Program to Engage Older Adults in Fall Prevention in a Nursing Home. *J. Nurs. Care Qual.* **2021**, 3 327–332. [CrossRef]
70. Tchouaket, É.; Kilpatrick, K.; Jabbour, M. Effectiveness for introducing nurse practitioners in six long-term care facilities i Québec, Canada: A cost-savings analysis. *Nurs. Outlook* **2020**, *68*, 611–625. [CrossRef]
71. Bourbonnais, A.; Rousseau, J.; Lalonde, M.H.; Meunier, J.; Lapierre, N.; Gagnon, M.P. Conditions and ethical challenges tha could influence the implementation of technologies in nursing homes: A qualitative study. *Int. J. Older People Nurs.* **2019**, *14* e12266. [CrossRef]
72. Choi, Y.; Staley, B.; Henriksen, C.; Xu, D.; Lipori, G.; Brumback, B.; Winterstein, A.G. A dynamic risk model for inpatient falls *Am. J. Health Syst. Pharm.* **2018**, *75*, 1293–1303. [CrossRef]
73. Hoe, J.; Profyri, E.; Kemp, C.; Manela, M.; Webster, L.; Anthony, J.; Costafreda, S.; Arrojo, F.; Souris, H.; Livingston, G. Risk assessment for people living with dementia: A systematic review. *Int. Psychogeriatr.* **2024**, *36*, 263–288. [CrossRef]
74. LeLaurin, J.H.; Shorr, R.I. Preventing Falls in Hospitalized Patients: State of the Science. *Clin. Geriatr. Med.* **2019**, *35*, 273–283 [CrossRef] [PubMed]
75. Park, S.H. Tools for assessing fall risk in the elderly: A systematic review and meta-analysis. *Aging Clin. Exp. Res.* **2018**, *30*, 1–16 [CrossRef] [PubMed]
76. Kim, Y.J.; Choi, K.O.; Cho, S.H.; Kim, S.J. Validity of the Morse Fall Scale and the Johns Hopkins Fall Risk Assessment Tool for fall risk assessment in an acute care setting. *J. Clin. Nurs.* **2022**, *31*, 3584–3594. [CrossRef] [PubMed]
77. Heikkilä, A.; Lehtonen, L.; Junttila, K. Consequences of Inpatient Falls in Acute Care: A Retrospective Register Study. *J. Patient Saf.* **2024**, *20*, 340–344. [CrossRef]
78. Kim, D.W.; Seo, J.; Kwon, S.; Park, C.M.; Han, C.; Kim, Y.; Yoon, D.; Kim, K.M. Integrating real-time location systems with electronic medical records: A machine learning approach for in-hospital fall risk prediction. *medRxiv* **2024**. [CrossRef]
79. Jahandideh, S.; Hutchinson, A.F.; Bucknall, T.K.; Considine, J.; Driscoll, A.; Manias, E.; Phillips, N.M.; Rasmussen, B.; Vos, N.; Hutchinson, A.M. Using machine learning models to predict falls in hospitalised adults. *Int. J. Med. Inform.* **2024**, *187*, 105436. [CrossRef]

Resnick, B.; Young, H.M.; Fick, D.M.; Kagan, S.H. Making care for older people the choice of nurses today, tomorrow, and forever. *Geriatr. Nurs.* **2022**, *46*, A1–A2. [CrossRef]
Lewis, S.R.; Griffin, X.L. Preventing falls in older people: The evidence for environmental interventions and why history matters. *Cochrane Database Syst. Rev.* **2023**, *3*, ED000162. [CrossRef]
National Institute on Aging. *Falls and Fractures in Older Adults: Causes and Prevention*; U.S. Department of Health and Human Services: Atlanta, GA, USA, 2024. Available online: https://www.nia.nih.gov/health/falls-and-falls-prevention/falls-and-fractures-older-adults-causes-and-prevention (accessed on 3 December 2024).
Dawson, R.; Suen, J.; Sherrington, C.; Kwok, W.; Pinheiro, M.B.; Haynes, A.; McLennan, C.; Sutcliffe, K.; Kneale, D.; Dyer, S. Effective fall prevention exercise in residential aged care: An intervention component analysis from an updated systematic review. *Br. J. Sports Med.* **2024**, *58*, 641–648. [CrossRef]
Dyer, S.M.; Suen, J.; Kwok, W.S.; Dawson, R.; McLennan, C.; Cameron, I.D.; Hill, K.D.; Sherrington, C. Exercise for falls prevention in aged care: Systematic review and trial endpoint meta-analyses. *Age Ageing* **2023**, *52*, afad217. [CrossRef] [PubMed]
Albasha, N.; Ahern, L.; O'Mahony, L.; McCullagh, R.; Cornally, N.; McHugh, S.; Timmons, S. Implementation strategies to support fall prevention interventions in long-term care facilities for older persons: A systematic review. *BMC Geriatr.* **2023**, *23*, 47. [CrossRef] [PubMed]
Nunan, S.; Brown Wilson, C.; Henwood, T.; Parker, D. Fall risk assessment tools for use among older adults in long-term care settings: A systematic review of the literature. *Australas. J. Ageing* **2018**, *37*, 23–33. [CrossRef] [PubMed]
Chen, S.; Kearns, W.D.; Fozard, J.L.; Li, M. Personalized fall risk assessment for long-term care services improvement. In Proceedings of the 2017 Annual Reliability and Maintainability Symposium (RAMS), Orlando, FL, USA, 23–26 January 2017.
Baethge, C.; Goldbeck-Wood, S.; Mertens, S. SANRA-a scale for the quality assessment of narrative review articles. *Res. Integr. Peer Rev.* **2019**, *4*, 5. [CrossRef] [PubMed]

healthcare MDPI

Article

Association between Falls, Fear of Falling and Depressive Symptoms in Community-Dwelling Older Adults

Maria Eduarda Armando Pereira [1], Gerson de Souza Santos [2], Clara Rabite de Almeida [3], Kethlyn Cristina Santos Nunes [3], Monalisa Claudia Maria da Silva [3], Helena José [4,5], Luís Sousa [4,6] and Luciano Magalhães Vitorino [1,*]

1 Faculty of Medicine of Itajubá, Itajubá 37502-138, MG, Brazil; mariaearmandop@gmail.com
2 Department of Medicine, Centro Universitário Ages, Paripiranga 48430-000, BA, Brazil; gerson.s.santos@ages.edu.br
3 Department of Nursing, Federal University of Juiz de Fora, Juiz de Fora 36036-900, MG, Brazil; clararabite95@gmail.com (C.R.d.A.); nunes.kethlyn@estudante.ufjf.br (K.C.S.N.); monalisa.silva@ufjf.br (M.C.M.d.S.)
4 Atlântica School of Health, 2730-036 Barcarena, Portugal; hjose@uatlantica.pt (H.J.); luismmsousa@gmail.com (L.S.)
5 Health Sciences Research Unit: Nursing (UICISA: E), Nursing School of Coimbra, 3004-011 Coimbra, Portugal
6 Comprehensive Health Research Centre, University of Évora, 7000-801 Évora, Portugal
* Correspondence: lucianoenf@yahoo.com.br

Abstract: Background: Longevity increases pose public health challenges, especially in managing falls and their psychological impacts on older adults. Limited evidence exists on the relationship between a fear of falling (FOF), previous falls, and depressive symptoms among community-dwelling older adults. Objective: To evaluate the association between falls, FOF, and depressive symptoms in community-dwelling older adults. Methods: This cross-sectional study, conducted in 2018, included 400 older adults from a Basic Health Unit in São Paulo, Brazil. The Geriatric Depression Scale (GDS-15) and the International Falls Efficacy Scale (FES-I) were used, along with self-report questionnaires on fall history. Linear and logistic regression were used to analyze the relationships between variables. Results: The mean age was 75.2 (SD = 8.53) years, with 63.2% being female. Depressive symptoms were observed in 18.3% of the participants, while 90.5% reported a fear of falling (FOF). More than half (63.0%) experienced falls, with 49.5% occurring in the last year. Factors such as the female gender, negative health perceptions, and functional dependence were associated with depressive symptoms. Adjusted analyses indicated that both a fear of falling (FOF) (B = 0.043; $p = 0.012$) and a history of falls (B = 0.725; $p = 0.015$) were associated with depressive symptoms. Conclusions: Falls, FOF, and depressive symptoms are interlinked among older adults, underscoring the need for targeted interventions to improve their mental and physical health.

Keywords: aged; older people; fear of falling; falls; depression

1. Introduction

The rapid increase in the older population poses significant challenges for healthcare professionals, researchers, and health systems worldwide. A major challenge is preserving the autonomy and quality of life (QoL) of this population, which is affected by the high incidence of chronic non-communicable diseases (CNCDs) [1]. Mental illnesses are a major type of chronic non-communicable disease (CNCD) that affect the quality of life (QoL) of older adults [2]. Frailty significantly elevates the risk of depression among older adults [3]. Additionally, falls represent a critical risk factor for mental health deterioration, as they are the leading cause of disability in this population [4,5]. A recent meta-analysis with 14 studies identified a strong relationship between falls (whether single or recurrent), or a fear of falling, and a higher risk of developing depression among older persons [6].

Depression is a debilitating condition that contributes to increased morbidity, mortality, and healthcare costs [7]. It affects a significant portion of the older population globally, with a prevalence of 35.1% worldwide and 40.8% in developing countries like Brazil. In Brazil, the average estimated prevalence of depressive symptoms among community-dwelling older persons is 21.0% [8,9]. A large European study with 67,603 participants, averaging 67.9 years in age, identified social isolation and a poorer self-assessment of one's health status as the two strongest predictors of depression. Additionally, limitations in instrumental activities of daily living were significant predictors of depression in men, while the family burden was significant for women. Furthermore, mobility difficulties were found to increase the risk of falls and fear of falling for both sexes [10]. A meta-analysis of 17 studies involving 15,491 Brazilian older persons identified being female and having cardiovascular diseases as significant risk factors for depression [11].

Among the older population, falls are directly associated with the fear of falling and vice versa [12]. Generally, there are two ways to describe the fear of falling. The first is the definition focused on the fear itself, measuring the fearful anticipation of future falls. While an activity avoided out of fear can protect one from dangerous situations, if it exceeds a certain level, it becomes debilitating, starting a vicious cycle of inactivity, followed by the loss of physical conditioning and decreased confidence and social activity participation, ultimately enhancing the factors that increase the risk of depressive symptoms among older persons [13]. A Korean longitudinal study with 2933 older persons and 22 years of follow-up identified that both older persons who fell and did not have physical limitations and those who fell and had physical limitations experienced a substantial increase in the risk of depression [14].

Although the links between depressive symptoms and the risk of falls are not fully understood, several explanations exist. The use of selective serotonin reuptake inhibitors (SSRIs) and serotonin–norepinephrine reuptake inhibitors (SNRIs) significantly increases the risk of falls and fear of falling among older persons [15,16]. These medications can cause sedation, impaired balance, hyponatremia, cardiac arrhythmia, and drug-induced parkinsonism [16]. Depressive symptoms are associated with risk factors for falls, such as psychomotor slowness, leading to reduced walking speeds and imbalance [6]. People with depression may exhibit postural irregularities and changes in gait patterns, suggesting physiological causes for falls [17]. Additionally, depressive symptoms are linked to cognitive impairments that decrease attention, executive performance, and processing agility, increasing the risk of falls [18]. Geriatric depression is also associated with reduced appetite, weight loss, and muscle mass loss, further elevating the risk of falling [19].

Compared to other chronic non-communicable diseases (CNCDs), the prevalence of depressive symptoms in older persons, particularly when associated with factors such as a fear of falling, is relatively underexplored, especially in Brazil, as well as worldwide. The global prevalence of the fear of falling is 49.60%, with higher rates in developing countries (53.40%) than in developed countries (46.7%) and higher in patients (52.20%) than in community residents (48.40%) [20]. Falls are a significant public health issue among older adults, with an estimated 684,000 fatal falls occurring annually, making them the second leading cause of unintentional injury deaths globally (World Health Organization, 2021) [19]. A review of 104 studies with 36,740,590 participants found the global prevalence of falls in older people to be 26.5% (95% CI 23.4–29.8%) [21].

Effective fall prevention strategies, including education, safer environments, and policy implementation, are crucial [19]. In hospital and residential environments, falls are frequent but are challenging to prevent. An Italian study showed varying compliance with guidelines, indicating a need for standardized fall management and prevention strategies [20]. The lack of comprehensive evidence on the intersection of depression, a fear of falling, and falls in older adults may lead to inconsistent and suboptimal care. Depression is often underdiagnosed and undertreated in primary care settings, highlighting the necessity of addressing these gaps to improve healthcare outcomes. Gambaro et al. [6] support the association between a fear of falling and depressive symptoms, showing that various pieces of epidemiological evidence link depressive symptoms in older adults to numerous risk factors for falls, including psychomotor delays that can reduce walking speeds and impair balance. Understanding these connections is crucial in improving QoL and promoting better aging among older adults.

Although there have been studies on this topic, to our knowledge, there are no studies focusing on community-dwelling older adults in Brazil using validated and reliable scales for the fear of falling and depressive symptoms. This would allow for meaningful comparisons and strengthen the practice of comprehensive geriatric assessment. The practical contributions of our study include offering valuable data that can inform healthcare policies and interventions aimed at improving the mental and physical health of older adults. Thus, this study aims to assess the association between falls, a fear of falling, and depressive symptoms among Brazilian community-dwelling older adults.

2. Materials and Methods

2.1. Study Design

This is a cross-sectional study that is part of a multidimensional study with older persons (aged 60 years or more) registered at a Basic Health Unit (BHU) in São Paulo, SP, Brazil. The study project was approved by the Research Ethics Committee of the Faculty of Medicine of Itajubá, (#2.468.315) on 17 January 2018. All participants signed an informed consent form.

2.2. Location and Sample

The study was conducted with older persons registered at the Marcus Belenzinho BHU located in the East Zone, the most populous area of São Paulo, SP. The sample size was calculated based on the following questions. (1) Would there be differences between the group of older persons who had a fear of falling and the group that did not have this fear regarding depressive symptoms? A meta-analysis showed a relative risk of 2.85 between a fear of falling and depression in the older population [6]. (2) Would there be differences between the group of older persons who had fallen in the last 12 months and the group that had not fallen in the last 12 months regarding depressive symptoms? A longitudinal study identified a risk of 2.73 between falling and depression [22]. The G*Power 3.1.9.7 program was used to calculate the statistical power of the analyses, with the aim of implementing multivariate linear and logistic regression models, with 3 independent variables (variables with $p < 0.10$ in bivariate analysis), with a relative risk of 2.85 between the fear of falling (considering the highest relative risk) and depressive symptoms, a two-tailed p-value, and 400 participants. The post hoc analysis showed the statistical power of the analyses to be 97.8%.

2.3. Data Collection and Inclusion and Exclusion Criteria

Data collection was conducted between February and August 2018 by a nurse during nursing consultations at the BHU, with an average duration of 40 minutes. Simple random sampling, based on the records of 5000 older persons registered at the BHU Marcus Belenzinho, was used to obtain the study participants. The inclusion criteria encompassed participants aged 60 years or older and registered at the BHU Belenzinho. Individuals with severe physical limitations (e.g., difficulty feeding themselves, bathing, or using the bathroom or severe respiratory difficulties) and a medical diagnosis of moderate to severe cognitive deficits or dementia were not included.

2.4. Measurement

Depressive Symptoms: The abbreviated Geriatric Depression Scale with 15 items (GDS-15) was used to investigate the participants' depressive symptoms. This scale was developed by Yesavage in 1983 [22] and validated in Portuguese in 2005 [23]. It is a fifteen-item scale, with two response options (yes; no). The score ranges from 0 to 15 and classifies patients without depressive symptoms (scores of 0 to 5) and with depressive symptoms (scores of 6 or greater) [22,23]. Example questions include "Are you satisfied with your life?" (yes/no), "Do you often feel helpless?" (yes/no), and "Do you feel your life is empty?" (yes/no). The sensitivity (86.5%) refers to the scale's ability to correctly identify those with depressive symptoms, while the specificity (63.3%) refers to the scale's ability to correctly identify those without depressive symptoms. In the Brazilian validation, the GDS-15 showed good reliability, with a Cronbach's alpha of 0.81 [24].

2.5. Data Collected

Fear of Falls: We used the Falls Efficacy Scale—International (FES-I), developed by Yardley in 2005 [25]. This scale was validated in 2010 for the Brazilian context [26]. The FES-I assesses the fear of falling in 16 different daily activities, including items such as moving into or out of a chair, walking in places with crowds, and cleaning the house (e.g., sweeping, vacuuming, dusting). The Falls Efficacy Scale—International (FES-I) scoring ranges from 16 (not concerned) to 64 (extremely concerned), with each item measured on a four-point Likert scale: 1 = not at all concerned, 2 = somewhat concerned, 3 = fairly concerned, and 4 = very concerned. The cutoff points for the fear of falling were as follows: 16–22 = low concern and 23–64 = high concern. In the Brazilian validation, the FES-I showed excellent reliability, with a Cronbach's alpha equal to 0.96 [26].

Fall History (self-report). To investigate the fall history in the last 12 months, the following question was asked: "Have you fallen at home, on the street, or elsewhere in the last 12 months?" (yes or no).

Sociodemographic Variables. We included the sociodemographic and health variables of the elderly participants, with notable divisions in each category. These included age (60–69, 70–79, and $\geq$80 years), gender (female and male), income (less than and more than 1 minimum wage), health status (poor to excellent), the presence of chronic diseases (yes and no), the daily use of medication (yes and no), polypharmacy (yes and no), functional independence according to the Katz Index of Activities of Daily Living (dependent and independent), functional independence according to the Lawton Instrumental Activities of Daily Living Scale (dependent and independent), fall history (have fallen and have never fallen), fear of falling (afraid and not afraid), and depressive symptoms (yes and no). This detailed structure provided a comprehensive basis for the analysis of the relationships between depression, the fear of falling, and the characteristics of the participants.

Basic activities of daily living were evaluated using the Katz Index, created by Sidney Katz in 1976 and validated in Portuguese in 2008 [27]. It is an instrument that assesses the basic activities of daily living (ADL) according to the degree of independence in the outcomes of six ADL functions (bathing, dressing, going to the toilet, transferring, continence, and feeding). Example questions include "Can you bathe yourself without assistance?" (yes/no), "Can you dress yourself without help?" (yes/no), and "Can you use the toilet independently?" (yes/no). The score ranges from 0 to 6 points and classifies patients as independent (score zero) and dependent (score greater than or equal to 1). Its reliability and internal consistency as assessed by Cronbach's alpha ranged from 0.80 to 0.92 [27].

Instrumental activities of daily living: Lawton Scale—devised by Lawton and Brody in 1969 and validated in Portuguese in 2008 [28]. It is used to assess the instrumental activities of daily living (IADL) according to scores ranging from 0 to 21. Example questions include "Can you prepare your own meals?" (yes/no), "Can you manage your own medications?" (yes/no), and "Can you handle your own finances?" (yes/no). It classifies patients as dependent (score less than or equal to 20) and independent (score equal to 21) [28]. The internal consistency measured according to Cronbach's alpha ranged from 0.90 to 0.93 [28] and the reproducibility was considered stable and objective [29].

2.6. Statistical Analysis

Data were analyzed using SPSS version 26 (SPSS Inc., Chicago, IL, USA), with all analyses conducted by the research coordinator, L.M.V. Descriptive statistics included absolute and relative values for categorical variables and measures of central tendency for continuous variables on the GDS-15 and FES-I scales.

For inferential analysis, we employed both linear and logistic regression models. First, simple linear regression was used to examine the association between depressive symptoms (GDS-15) and the fear of falling or fall history. Next, multiple linear regression was used to adjust the depressive symptoms for significant sociodemographic and health variables ($p < 0.05$)—specifically, gender, self-perception of health, and ADL.

The complete linear models employed were as follows.

Model 1: Depressive Symptoms = $\beta 0 + \beta 1 \times$ FES-I + ϵ.
Model 2: Depressive Symptoms = $\beta 0 + \beta 1 \times$ FES-I + $\beta 2 \times$ Gender + ϵ.
Model 3: Depressive Symptoms = $\beta 0 + \beta 1 \times$ FES-I + $\beta 2 \times$ Gender + $\beta 3 \times$ Self-Perception of Health Status + $\beta 4 \times$ ADL + ϵ.
Model 4: Depressive Symptoms = $\beta 0 + \beta 1 \times$ History of Falling + ϵ.
Model 5: Depressive Symptoms = $\beta 0 + \beta 1 \times$ History of Falling + $\beta 2 \times$ Gender + ϵ.
Model 6: Depressive Symptoms = $\beta 0 + \beta 1 \times$ History of Falling + $\beta 2 \times$ Gender + $\beta 3 \times$ Self-Perception of Health Status + $\beta 4 \times$ ADL + ϵ.

Finally, logistic regression models were utilized to analyze depressive symptoms (coded as 0 = without or 1 = with depressive symptoms) with independent variables such as a fear of falling or fall history, adjusting for the same covariates as in the multiple linear regression.

These models assessed the independent effects of a fear of falling and fall history on depressive symptoms, while controlling for sociodemographic and clinical variables. A significance level of 5.0% was set for all tests, with 95.0% confidence intervals.

3. Results

Out of the total of 488 participants invited to take part in this study, 400 completed all items of the questionnaires, 50 participants did not meet the inclusion criteria, and 38 refused to participate in the study. The sociodemographic and health characteristics are shown in Table 1. The average age of the participants was 75.2 (SD = 8.53) years; the majority were between 70 and 79 years old (39.8%) and female (63.2%), with poor/regular self-perceptions of health (62.6%) and with chronic diseases (92.2%). Regarding medication use, 90.7% of the participants used medication daily; of these, 37.0% exhibited polypharmacy ($\geq$5 medications/day). We identified that 27.0% of the participants were dependent on ADL and 39.5% on IADL. The majority of the older persons reported having suffered a fall (63.5%), with half of the falls occurring in the last year (49.5%). The majority of the older adults (90.5%) also exhibited a fear of falling (FES-I $\geq$ 23), while the prevalence of depressive symptoms (GDS $\geq$ 6) was 18.3%.

Table 1. Characterization of participants (N = 400).

Variable	n	%
Age		
60–69	104	26.0
70–79	159	39.8
≥80	137	34.2
Gender		
Female	253	63.2
Male	147	36.8
Family income		
<1 salary	51	12.8
>1 salary	349	87.2

Table 1. *Cont.*

Variable	n	%
Health status		
Awful	89	22.3
Regular	161	40.3
Good	120	30.0
Excellent	30	7.5
Chronic illness		
Yes	369	92.2
No	31	7.8
Medication use		
Yes	363	90.7
No	37	9.3
Polypharmacy		
Yes	148	37.0
No	252	63.0
BADL [1] (Katz)		
Dependent	108	27.0
Independent	292	73.0
IADL [2] (Lawton)		
Dependent	158	39.5
Indepentend	242	60.5
History of falls [3]		
Fell	252	63.0
Never fell	148	37.0
Last fall		
<1 year	198	49.5
>1 year	51	12.8
Never fell	151	37.8
Fear of falling (FES-1 [4])		
With fear (FES-I: 23–64)	362	90.5
Without fear (FES-I: 16–22)	38	9.5
Depressive symptoms		
Yes (GDS $\geq$ 6)	73	18.3
No (GDS $\leq$ 5)	327	81.8

[1] Basic Activities of Daily Living; [2] Instrumental Activities of Daily Living; [3] Last Year; [4] Falls Efficacy Scale—International.

Table 2 shows the mean scores of the FES-I scale and GDS-15.

Table 2. Fear of falling and depressive symptom scores of study participants (N = 400).

Variable	Mean (SD)	95% CI
Depressive Symptoms (GDS-15 [1])	5.98 (2.89)	5.72–6.28
Fear of Falling (FES-I [2])	41.84 (12.99)	40.65–43.10

(GDS $\geq$ 6) [1] Geriatric Depression Scale-15; [2] Falls Efficacy Scale—International.

Table 3 presents the results of the simple linear regression. Being female (B = −0.954; p = 0.002), having a worse perception of one's health (B = −0.555; p = 0.009), and being dependent for ADL (B = −0.893; p = 0.036) were associated with depressive symptoms.

The results of the adjusted linear regression are shown in Table 4. After adjusting for gender, the self-perception of one's health status, ADL, higher levels of fear of falling (B = 0.043; p = 0.012), and a history of falling (B = 0.725; p = 0.015) were associated with depressive symptoms.

Table 3. Associations between the independent variables and depressive symptoms among older participants (N = 400).

Variable	B (SE)	Beta	*p*-Value
Age (60–69)	−0.018 (0.023)	−0.054	0.427
Gender (female)	−0.954 (0.303)	−0.159	0.002
Family income (<1 minimum wage)	−0.105 (0.242)	−0.024	0.664
Health status (poor)	−0.555 (0.213)	−0.138	0.009
Chronic disease (yes)	−0.633 (1.002)	−0.059	0.528
Use of medications (yes)	−0.037 (0.927)	−0.004	0.968
Polypharmacy (yes)	0.247 (0.305)	−0.041	0.419
ADL [1] (dependent)	−0.893 (0.425)	−0.137	0.036
IADL [2] (dependent)	−0.170 (0.363)	−0.029	0.639

[1] Basic Activities of Daily Living; [2] Instrumental Activities of Daily Living.

Table 4. Associations between fear of falling and depressive symptoms adjusted for sociodemographic variables (N = 400).

Variable	B (SE)	Beta	*p*-Value	Adjusted R^2
FES-I [1] (average)	0.053 (0.011)	0.230	0.001	0.013
FES-I [1] (sociodemographic)	0.057 (0.016)	0.244	0.001	0.018
FES-I [1] (sociodemographic + clinical)	0.043 (0.17)	0.184	0.012	0.095
History of falling (yes)	1.017 (0.295)	0.170	0.001	0.027
History of falling (sociodemographic *)	0.853 (0.335)	0.143	0.011	0.130
History of falling (sociodemographic * + clinical)	0.725 (0.361)	0.188	0.015	0.150

[1] Falls Efficacy Scale—International. * Adjusted for sociodemographic (gender) and clinical (self-perception of health status and basic activities of daily living) variables.

The adjusted and unadjusted logistic regression (Table 5) indicated that older persons with a higher level of fear of falling (OR = 1.03, $p = 0.005$) and a history of falls (OR = 1.64, $p = 0.036$) showed a greater propensity for depressive symptoms.

Table 5. Unadjusted and adjusted logistic regression analyses between independent variables and depressive symptoms (N = 400).

Variable	OR (CI95%)	*p*-Value
FES-I [1] (average)	1.04 (1.022–1.05)	<0.001
FES-I [1] (sociodemographic)	1.03 (1.01–1.05)	0.001
FES-I [1] (sociodemographic + clinical)	1.03 (1.01–1.05)	0.005
History of falling (yes)	2.04 (1.34–3.09)	0.001
History of falling (sociodemographic *)	1.72 (1.11–2.67)	0.015
History of falling (sociodemographic * + clinical)	1.64 (1.03–2.62)	0.036

[1] Falls Efficacy Scale—International. * Adjusted for sociodemographic (gender) and clinical (self-perception of health status and basic activities of daily living) variables. GDS $\geq$ 6: Yes = 1; No = 0.

4. Discussion

This study explored how the fear of falling and a history of falls can impact mental health—specifically, depressive symptoms—in community-dwelling older persons. We identified that, after controlling for sociodemographic variables, an increase in the fear of falling and the presence of a history of falls were strongly associated with a higher prevalence of depressive symptoms. This finding is consistent with previous studies, such as a systematic review [8,23] and longitudinal research [24], reinforcing the relationship between these factors and depressive symptoms in older adults. In a meta-analysis that included 31 studies with 70,868 elderly people living in the community, the factors associated with falls were age, the female sex, a fear of falling, a history of falls, unclear vision, depression, and balance disorders [25]. A Greek study also found similar results and demonstrated that falling was associated with declining balance, depression, the female gender, and higher education [26]. However, a prospective study involving 6862 older people in Ireland found that falls increased the risk for incident symptoms of anxiety and depression [26].

We observed that a fear of falling among older adults is a prevalent reality that intensifies with age. This trend is influenced by both biological age and the subjective perception of one's age [27]. Our results point to a significant association between the fear of falls and the development of depressive symptoms. This relationship suggests that depressive symptoms may emerge as a direct consequence of social isolation and the loss of independence, both resulting from the limitations imposed by the fear of falls [6,28]. In a study involving 3443 individuals, poorer social engagement and network contact were found to be associated with a higher likelihood of falls, while a poorer neighborhood context was associated with a higher likelihood of fall injuries. Furthermore, social engagement mediated a significant portion of the effect of depression on the occurrence of falls, and the neighborhood context mediated a portion of the effect of depression on fall injuries [29].

Conversely, depression itself can exacerbate the fear of falling by reducing older adults' confidence in their physical abilities, creating a vicious cycle that affects both mental and physical health [6]. In a study conducted in Brazil, it was found that being a woman and having a higher number of self-reported morbidities, worse physical performance, and a higher number of depressive symptoms were associated with a higher level of fear of falling. In addition, it was found that physical inactivity, mediated by a higher number of morbidities, worse physical performance, and a higher number of depressive symptoms, was associated with a higher level of fear of falling [30]. Living arrangements, such as living alone, with family, or in an elderly home, can significantly influence these dynamics. For instance, living alone may increase the risk of social isolation and falls, while living with family can provide support but also create a potential family burden [12,31].

A scoping review covering 46 studies, supplemented by a Korean longitudinal study with 62,363 participants over 16 years, highlighted the complex interrelation between FOF and depressive symptoms in older adults [32,33]. The finding of an association between a fear of falling and depressive symptoms in 95% (19/20) of the studies analyzed in the scoping review underscores the association between a fear of falling and depressive symptoms. This phenomenon highlights that depression is not merely a psycho-emotional aspect of the fear of falling but also a factor that intensifies the associated risks, suggesting a vicious cycle where the fear of falling and depression are mutually intensified, exacerbating frailty and increasing the vulnerability of older adults. These findings underscore the urgent need for therapeutic approaches that encompass both mental health treatment and fall prevention strategies, aiming to mitigate this risk in the older population. Such approaches could include cognitive–behavioral therapy (CBT) to address both depression and the fear of falling, tailored physical exercise programs like Tai Chi and strength training to improve balance and confidence, and multifactorial interventions that combine medical, psychological, and physical therapy to meet the comprehensive needs of older adults. These interventions should be designed to reduce both the fear of falling and depressive symptoms, thereby improving the overall quality of life [31].

Our findings also reinforce the link between a history of falls and depressive symptoms in older adults, in line with previous studies. The systematic review by Xu et al. highlights depression as a significant risk factor for falls (RR 4.34) [34], surpassing other common conditions such as heart disease and hypertension. Factors related to depression, such as social isolation, apathy, physical inactivity, physical impairment, and the use of antidepressants, increase the risk of falls.

The relationship between depressive symptoms and falls, although well established, reveals complexities yet to be unraveled. Risk factors for falls, such as psychomotor delays, are associated with depressive symptoms, affecting individuals' locomotion speeds and balance. Gambaro et al. [6] underline a growing interest in the interaction between depression, falls, and a fear of falling, evidencing a bidirectional relationship: falls negatively affect independence and well-being, while depression can lead to psychomotor delays and changes in posture and gait. A longitudinal study in Korea showed a significant correlation between depressive symptoms and the number of previous falls, with depression remaining a risk factor even after adjusting for other variables, including the fear of falling [32].

4.1. Study Limitations and Strengths

While addressing the relationship between a fear of falling, a history of falls, and depressive symptoms in older adults, this study provides significant findings but also presents some important limitations that should be considered. Firstly, the cross-sectional nature of the study limits the ability to establish causal relationships between the variables. Additionally, factors such as financial issues, the family history, the home environmental conditions, and pre-existing diseases were not associated with the outcomes but could offer a deeper understanding of the dynamics at play. Another limitation is the participant group, which, although extensive, may not fully represent the diversity of the Brazilian older population, particularly in different cultural and socioeconomic contexts. This introduces a potential selection bias, as the sample was drawn from older persons registered at a BHU in São Paulo, Brazil and may not be representative of the Brazilian population of older adults. Future studies should aim to include a more representative sample to enhance the external validity of the findings.

Furthermore, the low adjusted R^2 values in our regression models indicate that, while the predictors are statistically significant, they explain only a small portion of the variance in depressive symptoms. This suggests that other factors, not included in our models, also contribute to depressive symptoms among older adults. The complexity of depressive symptoms, which are influenced by a wide range of biological, psychological, and social factors, could account for the relatively low explanatory power of our models.

However, the study also has strengths that should be highlighted. It includes a considerable sample of older adults, of both sexes and with varied socioeconomic conditions, enriching the analysis and allowing for a more comprehensive understanding of the factors associated with depressive symptoms in older adults. Moreover, the use of validated instruments, such as the Geriatric Depression Scale (GDS-15) and the Falls Efficacy Scale—International (FES-I), lends methodological robustness to the findings.

4.2. Implications for Clinical Practice, Policy, and Education

The results of this study are significant for healthcare professionals, especially in geriatrics, gerontology, and primary healthcare. With the increasing older population, managing the fear of falling and preventing falls to reduce depressive symptoms and improve the well-being of older adults is vital. The research emphasizes the importance of comprehensive geriatric assessments that consider the fear of falling, fall prevention, and depressive symptoms as key elements of older adult health.

For professionals in primary care, the findings highlight the need for preventive approaches. The risk of falling can be reduced by implementing exercise programs focused on balance and strength training, combining interventions targeting modifiable risk factors [35], as well as interventions to mitigate the fear of falling [36]. In a review of fall risk assessment instruments, 38 instruments were identified, with 23 tools targeting hospitalized patients, eight aimed at risk assessment in home residents, and seven that can be applied in both contexts. In this review, the FES-I is recommended for the assessment of the fear of falling. However, as the nature of the fall risk is multifactorial, there is no "ideal" instrument in this sense. It is recommended to apply a combination of instruments, associated with direct and in-depth analysis carried out by the health professional [37].

Taking into account the above, implementing screening programs and interventions to identify and treat the fear of falls early is crucial to avoid negative consequences such as social isolation and a loss of independence. A fear of falling can significantly influence physical function in older adults and consequently increase the risk of future falls. Therefore, healthcare professionals should assess the fear of falling and consider implementing strategies to reduce the fear of falling as part of a comprehensive, person-centered care plan [38]. These programs must have psycho-educational interventions that allow the empowerment and training of the older adult and their family caregiver/informal caregiver, in self-care and activities of daily living, as well as in physical exercise (Tai Chi, yoga, balance training, or strength and resistance training) and fall prevention [39–42].

Integrating these assessments into regular care would help to promote the health of older adults and prevent mental and physical health problems. These interventions regarding the prevention of the risk of falling and fear of falling must be based on the policies of the World Health Organization, which aim to contribute to healthy aging, in order to prevent diseases, promote physical and mental health, and maintain functional capacity [43].

These results also have implications for education policies. In this sense, modules on assessment and intervention aimed at preventing the risk of falls, fear of falling, and depressive symptoms in community-dwelling older adults should be integrated into undergraduate and postgraduate courses, in lectures or modules on physical exercise prescription and physical activity in elderly people. With better-prepared professionals, this will contribute to safer and more person-centered care.

5. Conclusions

A fear of falling, a history of falls, and depressive symptoms are complex and interconnected factors that have a significant impact on the lives of older people. Previous research indicates that a fear of falling is often associated with previous falls and can lead to adverse consequences such as restricted physical activity and a loss of functional independence, and the experience of falls is often followed by physical and emotional complications, with potential sequelae ranging from physical injuries to the development of mental disorders such as depression.

Our findings establish a significant association between the fear of falling, a history of falls, and depressive symptoms among older people, highlighting their high prevalence and negative impact on mental health. These results underscore the importance of developing integrated strategies focused on fall prevention, managing the fear of falling, and treating depression, aimed at enhancing the physical and mental health of this population. It is undeniable that the relationship between falls, a fear of falling, and depressive symptoms in older people is a crucial area of research, requiring holistic and personalized interventions to improve the health and well-being of this vulnerable population.

Author Contributions: Conceptualization, L.M.V., G.d.S.S. and M.E.A.P.; methodology, L.M.V., G.d.S.S., M.E.A.P., C.R.d.A., K.C.S.N. and M.C.M.d.S.; software, L.M.V.; validation, L.M.V. and L.S.; formal analysis, L.M.V.; investigation, G.d.S.S.; resources, L.M.V., G.d.S.S., M.E.A.P., C.R.d.A., K.C.S.N. and M.C.M.d.S.; data curation, L.M.V. and G.d.S.S.; writing—original draft preparation, L.M.V., G.d.S.S., M.E.A.P., C.R.d.A., K.C.S.N., M.C.M.d.S., H.J. and L.S.; writing—review and editing, L.M.V., G.d.S.S., M.E.A.P., C.R.d.A., K.C.S.N., M.C.M.d.S., H.J. and L.S.; visualization, L.M.V., G.d.S.S., M.E.A.P., C.R.d.A., K.C.S.N., M.C.M.d.S., H.J. and L.S.; supervision, L.M.V.; project administration, L.M.V. and G.d.S.S. All authors have read and agreed to the published version of the manuscript.

Funding: This research received no external funding.

Institutional Review Board Statement: The study was conducted in accordance with the Declaration of Helsinki and approved by the Research Ethics Committee of the Faculty of Medicine of Itajubá (#2.468.315) on 17 January 2018.

Informed Consent Statement: Informed consent was obtained from all subjects involved in the study.

Data Availability Statement: Data will be available upon request (lucianoenf@yahoo.com.br).

Conflicts of Interest: The authors declare no conflicts of interest.

References

1. Prince, M.J.; Wu, F.; Guo, Y.; Gutierrez Robledo, L.M.; O'Donnell, M.; Sullivan, R.; Yusuf, S. The burden of disease in older peo and implications for health policy and practice. *Lancet* **2015**, *385*, 549–562. [CrossRef] [PubMed]
2. Scherrer, G., Jr.; Passos, K.G.; Oliveira, L.M.d.; Okuno, M.F.P.; Alonso, A.C.; Belasco, A.G.S. Atividades de vida diária, sinto depressivos e qualidade de vida de idosos. *Acta Paul. Enferm.* **2022**, *35*, eAPE0237345. [CrossRef]
3. Nascimento, P.P.P.d.; Aprahamian, I.; Yassuda, M.S.; Neri, A.L.; Batistoni, S.S.T. Fragilidade, depressão e mortalidade em u coorte de pessoas idosas residentes na comunidade. *Rev. Bras. Geriatr. Gerontol.* **2022**, *25*, e210225. [CrossRef]
4. Park, Y.; Paik, N.J.; Kim, K.W.; Jang, H.C.; Lim, J.Y. Depressive Symptoms, Falls, and Fear of Falling in Old Korean Adults: T Korean Longitudinal Study on Health and Aging (KLoSHA). *J. Frailty Aging* **2017**, *6*, 144–147. [CrossRef] [PubMed]
5. Zhang, Q.; Zhao, X.; Liu, H.; Ding, H. Frailty as a predictor of future falls and disability: A four-year follow-up study of Chine older adults. *BMC Geriatr.* **2020**, *20*, 388. [CrossRef] [PubMed]
6. Gambaro, E.; Gramaglia, C.; Azzolina, D.; Campani, D.; Molin, A.D.; Zeppegno, P. The complex associations between late li depression, fear of falling and risk of falls. A systematic review and meta-analysis. *Ageing Res. Rev.* **2022**, *73*, 101532. [CrossRe [PubMed]
7. König, H.; König, H.H.; Konnopka, A. The excess costs of depression: A systematic review and meta-analysis. *Epidemiol. Psychia Sci.* **2019**, *29*, e30. [CrossRef] [PubMed]
8. Cai, H.; Jin, Y.; Liu, R.; Zhang, Q.; Su, Z.; Ungvari, G.S.; Tang, Y.L.; Ng, C.H.; Li, X.H.; Xiang, Y.T. Global prevalence of depressic in older adults: A systematic review and meta-analysis of epidemiological surveys. *Asian J. Psychiatr.* **2023**, *80*, 103417. [CrossRe [PubMed]
9. Meneguci, J.; Meneguci, C.A.G.; Moreira, M.M.; Pereira, K.R.; Tribess, S.; Sasaki, J.E.; Virtuoso Júnior, J.S. Prevalência d sintomatologia depressiva em idosos brasileiros: Uma revisão sistemática com metanálise. *J. Bras. Psiquiatr.* **2019**, *68*, 221–2 [CrossRef]
10. Handing, E.P.; Strobl, C.; Jiao, Y.; Feliciano, L.; Aichele, S. Predictors of depression among middle-aged and older men an women in Europe: A machine learning approach. *Lancet Reg. Health Eur.* **2022**, *18*, 100391. [CrossRef]
11. Barcelos-Ferreira, R.; Izbicki, R.; Steffens, D.C.; Bottino, C.M. Depressive morbidity and gender in community-dwelling Brazilia elderly: Systematic review and meta-analysis. *Int. Psychogeriatr.* **2010**, *22*, 712–726. [CrossRef]
12. Lavedán, A.; Viladrosa, M.; Jürschik, P.; Botigué, T.; Nuín, C.; Masot, O.; Lavedán, R. Fear of falling in community-dwelling old adults: A cause of falls, a consequence, or both? *PLoS ONE* **2018**, *13*, e0194967. [CrossRef]
13. Rakhshani, T.; Ansari, M.H.; Ebrahimi, M.; Ebrahimi, M.R.; Pearson, S.K. Fear of falling and its association with anxiety an depression disorders among community-dwelling older adults. *Int. J. Health Promot. Educ.* **2019**, *57*, 303–315. [CrossRef]
14. Lee, T.H.; Kim, W. Is fear of falling and the associated restrictions in daily activity related to depressive symptoms in older adults *Psychogeriatrics* **2021**, *21*, 304–310. [CrossRef] [PubMed]
15. Haddad, Y.K.; Luo, F.; Bergen, G.; Legha, J.K.; Atherly, A. Special Report from the CDC Antidepressant subclass use and fall ris in community-dwelling older Americans. *J. Saf. Res.* **2021**, *76*, 332–340. [CrossRef] [PubMed]
16. van Poelgeest, E.P.; Pronk, A.C.; Rhebergen, D.; van der Velde, N. Depression, antidepressants and fall risk: Therapeuti dilemmas-a clinical review. *Eur. Geriatr. Med.* **2021**, *12*, 585–596. [CrossRef]
17. Lenardt, M.H.; Falcão, A.d.S.; Hammerschmidt, K.S.d.A.; Barbiero, M.M.A.; Leta, P.R.G.; Sousa, R.L.d. Sintomas depressivos fragilidade física em pessoas idosas: Revisão integrativa. *Rev. Bras. Geriatr. Gerontol.* **2021**, *24*, e210013. [CrossRef]
18. Montero-Odasso, M.; Speechley, M. Falls in Cognitively Impaired Older Adults: Implications for Risk Assessment and Preventior *J. Am. Geriatr. Soc.* **2018**, *66*, 367–375. [CrossRef]
19. Gao, Q.; Hu, K.; Yan, C.; Zhao, B.; Mei, F.; Chen, F.; Zhao, L.; Shang, Y.; Ma, Y.; Ma, B. Associated Factors of Sarcopenia i Community-Dwelling Older Adults: A Systematic Review and Meta-Analysis. *Nutrients* **2021**, *13*, 4291. [CrossRef]
20. Xiong, W.; Wang, D.; Ren, W.; Liu, X.; Wen, R.; Luo, Y. The global prevalence of and risk factors for fear of falling among olde adults: A systematic review and meta-analysis. *BMC Geriatr.* **2024**, *24*, 321. [CrossRef]
21. Salari, N.; Darvishi, N.; Ahmadipanah, M.; Shohaimi, S.; Mohammadi, M. Global prevalence of falls in the older adults: A comprehensive systematic review and meta-analysis. *J. Orthop. Surg. Res.* **2022**, *17*, 334. [CrossRef]
22. Choi, N.G.; Marti, C.N.; DiNitto, D.M.; Kunik, M.E. Longitudinal Associations of Falls and Depressive Symptoms in Older Adults *Gerontologist* **2019**, *59*, 1141–1151. [CrossRef]
23. Brasileiro, L.E.E.; Paiva, A.L.M.; de Medeiros, M.Y.D.; Jerez-Roig, J.; de Souza, D.L.B. Incidence of depression and depressive symptoms and their predictive factors in community-dwelling older adults: A systematic review and meta-analysis protocol *BMJ Open* **2021**, *11*, e052147. [CrossRef]
24. de la Torre-Luque, A.; Ayuso-Mateos, J.L. The course of depression in late life: A longitudinal perspective. *Epidemiol. Psychiatr. Sci.* **2020**, *29*, e147. [CrossRef] [PubMed]
25. Li, Y.; Hou, L.; Zhao, H.; Xie, R.; Yi, Y.; Ding, X. Risk factors for falls among community-dwelling older adults: A systematic review and meta-analysis. *Front. Med.* **2022**, *9*, 1019094. [CrossRef]
26. Jacob, L.; Kostev, K.; Shin, J.I.; Smith, L.; Oh, H.; Abduljabbar, A.S.; Haro, J.M.; Koyanagi, A. Falls increase the risk for incident anxiety and depressive symptoms among adults aged ≥50 years: An analysis of the Irish longitudinal study on ageing. *Arch. Gerontol. Geriatr.* **2023**, *114*, 105098. [CrossRef] [PubMed]

Fundenberger, H.; Stephan, Y.; Hupin, D.; Barth, N.; Terracciano, A.; Canada, B. Prospective associations between subjective age and fear of falling in older adults. *Aging Ment. Health* **2022**, *26*, 86–91. [CrossRef]

Kupferberg, A.; Hasler, G. The social cost of depression: Investigating the impact of impaired social emotion regulation, social cognition, and interpersonal behavior on social functioning. *J. Affect. Disord. Rep.* **2023**, *14*, 100631. [CrossRef]

Lohman, M.C.; Fallahi, A.; Mishio Bawa, E.; Wei, J.; Merchant, A.T. Social Mediators of the Association Between Depression and Falls Among Older Adults. *J. Aging Health* **2023**, *35*, 593–603. [CrossRef]

dos Santos, E.P.R.; Ohara, D.G.; Patrizzi, L.J.; de Walsh, I.A.P.; Silva, C.d.F.R.; da Silva Neto, J.R.; Oliveira, N.G.N.; Matos, A.P.; Iosimuta, N.C.R.; Pinto, A.C.P.N.; et al. Investigating Factors Associated with Fear of Falling in Community-Dwelling Older Adults through Structural Equation Modeling Analysis: A Cross-Sectional Study. *J. Clin. Med.* **2023**, *12*, 545. [CrossRef]

Stubbs, B.; Brefka, S.; Denkinger, M.D. What Works to Prevent Falls in Community-Dwelling Older Adults? Umbrella Review of Meta-analyses of Randomized Controlled Trials. *Phys. Ther.* **2015**, *95*, 1095–1110. [CrossRef]

Yao, S.; Chen, X.W. The association between depressive symptoms with fear of falling and cognitive decline in older adults in the Korean community: An analysis of the Korean Longitudinal Study of Aging (KLoSA), 2006–2020. *Arch. Gerontol. Geriatr.* **2024**, *117*, 105177. [CrossRef] [PubMed]

MacKay, S.; Ebert, P.; Harbidge, C.; Hogan, D.B. Fear of Falling in Older Adults: A Scoping Review of Recent Literature. *Can. Geriatr. J.* **2021**, *24*, 379–394. [CrossRef] [PubMed]

Xu, Q.; Ou, X.; Li, J. The risk of falls among the aging population: A systematic review and meta-analysis. *Front. Public Health* **2022**, *10*, 902599. [CrossRef] [PubMed]

Sousa, L.; Tomás, J.; Severino, S.; Valido, S.; Santos, M.J.; José, H. Preventing falls in the aged: A challenge in patient safety. *Salud Cienc. Tecnol.* **2024**, *4*, 1000. [CrossRef]

Hawkins, M.; Goldhammer, T.; McClave, R.; Jenkins-Smith, E. Evaluation of a Fall Prevention Program to Reduce Fall Risk and Fear of Falling Among Community-Dwelling Older Adults and Adults with Disabilities. *Clin. Interv. Aging* **2024**, *19*, 375–383. [CrossRef]

Strini, V.; Schiavolin, R.; Prendin, A. Fall Risk Assessment Scales: A Systematic Literature Review. *Nurs. Rep.* **2021**, *11*, 430–443. [CrossRef]

Whipple, M.O.; Hamel, A.V.; Talley, K.M.C. Fear of falling among community-dwelling older adults: A scoping review to identify effective evidence-based interventions. *Geriatr. Nurs.* **2018**, *39*, 170–177. [CrossRef]

Ferreira, R.; Pedrosa, A.R.; Reis, N.; Sousa, L.; Nicolau, C.; Ferreira, B.; Rocha, B.; Baixinho, C.L. Transitional care for older persons with need of geriatric rehabilitation nursing interventions. *BMC Nurs.* **2024**, *23*, 376. [CrossRef]

Gemito, L.; Alves, E.; Moreira, J.; Marques, M.F.; Caldeira, E.; Ferreira, R.; Bico, I.; Pinho, L.; Fonseca, C.; Sousa, L.; et al. Programmes Addressed to Informal Caregivers' Needs: A Systematic Literature Review. *Geriatrics* **2024**, *9*, 71. [CrossRef]

Sadaqa, M.; Németh, Z.; Makai, A.; Prémusz, V.; Hock, M. Effectiveness of exercise interventions on fall prevention in ambulatory community-dwelling older adults: A systematic review with narrative synthesis. *Front. Public Health* **2023**, *11*, 1209319. [CrossRef] [PubMed]

Yoshikawa, A.; Ramirez, G.; Smith, M.L.; Lee, S.; Ory, M.G. Systematic Review and Meta-Analysis of Fear of Falling and Fall-Related Efficacy in a Widely Disseminated Community-Based Fall Prevention Program. *Arch. Gerontol. Geriatr.* **2020**, *91*, 104235. [CrossRef] [PubMed]

WHO's Work on the UN Decade of Healthy Ageing: Plan of Action (2021–2030); WHO: Geneva, Switzerland, 2020.

healthcare

MDPI

Article

Association between Polypharmacy and Hospitalization among Older Adults Admitted to Emergency Departments for Falls in Guadeloupe: A Retrospective Cohort Study

Nadine Simo-Tabue [1,2], Laurys Letchimy [3,4], Ludwig Mounsamy [5], Leila Rinaldo [5], Larissa Vainqueur [5], Marie-Josiane Ntsama-Essomba [6], Guillaume Mallet [5], Denis Boucaud-Maitre [7,8] and Maturín Tabue Teguo [1,9,10,*]

1 Unité de Recherche EpiCliV, Université des Antilles, 97233 Fort-de-France, France
2 Service de Gériatrie, CHU de Martinique, 97261 Fort-de-France, France
3 Pôle Gériatrie-Gérontologie, Université des Antilles, 97233 Fort-de-France, France
4 CHU de Martinique, 97261 Fort-de-France, France
5 CHU Pointe à Pitre, Université des Antilles, 97233 Fort-de-France, France; ludwig.mounsamy@chu-guadeloupe.fr (L.M.)
6 Hôpital Central de Yaoundé, Yaoundé P.O. Box 25625, Cameroon; ebomaj2012@gmail.com
7 Centre Hospitalier le Vinatier, 69500 Bron, France
8 Epidémiologie Clinique et Vieillissement (EpiCliV), Université des Antilles, 97233 Fort-de-France, France
9 Département de Recherche Clinique et Innovation, CHU de Martinique, 97261 Fort-de-France, France
10 Equipe ACTIVE, Université de Bordeaux, 33405 Talence, France
* Correspondence: tabue.maturin@gmail.com

Abstract: Introduction: Falls are a common geriatric syndrome in older people. Falls are associated with adverse health events such as dependency, unplanned emergency admissions and death. This study aimed to identify the factors associated with fall severity, such as diabetes, hypertension, heart disease, cognitive decline and polypharmacy, as well as sociodemographic characteristics in patients aged 70 years and over admitted to the emergency department in Guadeloupe. **Method:** A single-center, observational, retrospective study of patients aged 70 years and over admitted to the emergency department (ED) of the University Hospital of Guadeloupe for a fall between 1 May 2018 and 30 April 2019 was conducted. Fall severity was defined as the need for hospitalization. Bivariate analysis was used to determine the associations between fall severity and sociodemographic characteristics, comorbidities, history of falls and polypharmacy (defined as the daily use of at least five drugs). Polypharmacy was analyzed as a binary variable (>5 drugs daily; yes or no) in categories (0–3 (ref.), 4–6, 7–9 and ≥10 drugs). **Results:** During the study period, 625 patients who attended the ED for a fall were included. The mean age was 82.6 ± 7.6 years, and 51.2% were women. Of these, 277 patients (44.3%) were admitted to the hospital, and 3 patients (0.5%) died. In the bivariate analysis, only polypharmacy was associated with hospitalization for a fall (OR: 1.63 [95% CI: 1.33–2.02]). The odds ratios for the polypharmacy categories were 1.46 [95% CI 0.99–2.14], 1.65 [1.09–2.50] and 1.48 [0.76–2.85] for 4–6, 7–9 and ≥10 drugs, respectively. **Conclusions:** Polypharmacy was associated with hospitalization as a proxy for fall severity. A regular review of drug prescriptions is essential to reduce polypharmacy in older adults.

Keywords: fall; elderly; Guadeloupe; emergency

1. Introduction

Falls are a common geriatric syndrome in older people [1,2]. A fall is defined as any involuntary event that causes the person to come to rest on the ground or at a lower level than the starting position without being the result of an acute incident such as a stroke [3]. Falls predict adverse health events, such as the need for admission to a nursing home, attendance at an emergency department (ED) and death [4]. The mortality rate attributable to falls among older people in the community is estimated at 5%, corresponding to around 9000 deaths per year among people aged 75 years and over in France. The annual risk of hospitalization due to falls is estimated to be 20% [5]. Falls are furthermore associated with a reduction in the quality of life [6–8], and are costly from a medico-economic perspective [9].

Several studies have focused on preventing falls in older people [10] in the community [11] or in nursing home [12] and hospital [13] settings. In a review of the literature on interventions to reduce falls in older people in hospital, Morris et al. showed that falls in hospitals can be prevented mainly by training healthcare professionals and raising their awareness [3]. Numerous interventions have been shown to be effective in preventing falls [14–17]. In a recent study carried out in Portugal in 2021, the authors investigated hospital admissions due to falls and found that they accounted for 2.1% of the total number of hospital admissions over a period of 9 years [18]. Vu et al. found a high prevalence of recurrent falls among older people hospitalized due to fall injuries in Vietnam [19]. Polymedication is a common geriatric syndrome among the elderly [20]. It is defined as "the simultaneous administration of many drugs or the administration of an excessive number of drugs". It is estimated that between 14% and 49% of patients aged over 75 take more than five medications a day [21]. As with falls, it is linked to adverse health outcomes, including mortality, hospitalization and falls [22]. The risk of falling increases with each new treatment prescribed [23].

To the best of our knowledge, in the Caribbean region [24–26], and in Guadeloupe in particular [27], very few studies have investigated falls and fall severity in the region. The aim of this study was therefore to identify the factors associated with fall severity (as assessed by need for hospitalization) in patients aged 70 years and over attending the emergency department in Guadeloupe.

2. Methods

2.1. Study Design

Setting: This was a retrospective, observational, single-center study of older adults in the emergency department of the University Hospital of Guadeloupe.

Setting: In this region of almost 380,000 inhabitants, there are three emergency departments (ED), one in the private sector and two in the public sector. The emergency department of the University Hospital of Guadeloupe accounts for 2/3 of all stays in the region. Therefore, only this ED participated in this study from 1 May 2018 to 30 April 2019 (i.e., prior to the start of the COVID-19 pandemic).

Participants: All patients aged 70 years and older who attended the ED because of a fall were identified from the hospital informatics database. The keywords used were "fall" ("fell/fallen").

Inclusion criteria: The inclusion criteria were as follows: age $\geq$ 70 years, fall as the reason for consultation and a completed entry prescription.

Exclusion criteria: Patients were excluded from the study if their entry prescription was incomplete or could not be found.

Ethical issue: All patients admitted to the emergency department of the University Hospital Center were informed that their data may be used for research purposes. Informed consent was obtained from all subjects and/or their legal guardian(s). All participants and their representatives were informed about the study by the investigators and were given the opportunity to specifically opt out of the use of their medical data for research purposes. Those who expressed opposition were not recruited. The research was carried out using Resurgence* computer software (https://www.resurgencecomputers.com/home), which is used on a daily basis in the emergency department. In compliance with the Declaration of Helsinki and French data protection laws, the study protocol was approved by the Ethics Committee of the University Hospital of Guadeloupe on 25 August 2019. All methods were applied in accordance with applicable guidelines and regulations.

2.2. Outcome Measure

The outcome of interest was fall severity, defined as the need for hospital admission from the ED.

2.3. Other Variables

Sociodemographic characteristics (age and sex); presence of chronic diseases and/or geriatric syndromes (hypertension, diabetes, cognitive disorders and history of falls in the past 12 months); functional status (dependence); place of residence (nursing home, at home or foster family); chronic/acute alcohol use and ongoing medication were also recorded.

2.4. Statistical Analysis

Quantitative variables are expressed as the mean ± standard deviation and categorical variables as percentage. Ongoing medications were grouped by International Common Denomination and then counted. Dependency was classified into two categories: totally dependent versus not totally dependent. The polypharmacy variable was considered first in binary form (>5 drugs daily; yes or no) and in categories (0–3 (reference), 4–6, 7–9 and ≥10 drugs). Bivariate logistic regression analyses were performed to investigate the relationship between fall severity and each variable. p-values < 0.05 were considered statistically significant. All analyses were conducted using R.3.0.2.

3. Results

A total of 813 patients attended the ED of the CHU of Guadeloupe for falls during the study period. After the exclusion of duplicates and false positives, 658 patients were eligible for the study. For thirty-three people, we were unable to retrieve treatment orders. Finally, 625 patients were included in the study. The mean age of the participants was 82.6 ± 7.7 years, and 51.2% were women. In total, 277 patients (44.3%) required hospital admission, while the remaining 348 (55.7%) were discharged home. Three patients (0.5%) died in the ED after admission. For the outcomes of the remaining 274 patients, 181 (66.1%) were admitted to a medical ward and 93 (33.9%) were admitted to a surgical ward.

A total of 248 patients (39.7%) had polypharmacy (>5 drugs daily). In total, 32.5% had diabetes, 66.9% had hypertension, 19.5% had cognitive decline, 7.5% consumed alcohol and 7.4% had severe dependency (Table 1). Thirty-three patients were living in a nursing home or foster families. A quarter of the patients had a history of at least two falls in the previous year.

Table 1. Comparison of clinical characteristics of patients with and without hospitalization following a fall.

Variable	Overall N = 625	Admitted n = 277	Not Admitted n = 348	OR (95% CI)	p-Value
Age (years ± SD)	82.6 ± 7.7	82.4 ± 7.2	82.8 ± 8.1		0.522
Female, n (%)	320 (51.2%)	138 (49.8%)	182 (52.3%)		0.538
Institutionalized, n (%)	33 (5.3%)	14 (5.1%)	19 (5.5%)		0.821
Not totally dependent	579 (92.6%)	255 (92.1%)	324 (93.1%)		0.619
Diabetes	203 (32.5%)	90 (32.5%)	113 (32.5%)		0.996
Hypertension	418 (66.9%)	186 (67.2%)	232 (66.7%)		0.899
Heart disease	84 (13.4%)	42 (15.2%)	42 (12.1%)		0.260
Alcohol	47 (7.5%)	18 (6.5%)	29 (8.3%)		0.387
Stroke	81 (13.0%)	35 (12.6%)	46 (13.2%)		0.829
Epilepsy	34 (5.4%)	11 (4.0%)	23 (6.1%)		0.149

Table 1. *Cont.*

Variable	Overall N = 625	Admitted n = 277	Not Admitted n = 348	OR (95% CI)	*p*-Value
Parkinson	39 (6.2%)	16 (5.8%)	23 (6.6%)		0.669
Cognitive decline	122 (19.5%)	53 (19.1%)	69 (19.8%)		0.828
History of falls					
<2 in the previous year, n (%)	472 (75.5%)	210 (75.8%)	262 (75.3%)		0.879
2 in the previous per year, n (%)	153 (24.5%)	67 (24.2%)	86 (24.7%)		
'olypharmacy (>5 drugs), n (%)	248 (39.7%)	134 (48.4%)	114 (32.8%)	1.63 [1.33–2.02]	<0.001
Duration of stay in ED (hours ± SD)	10.4 ± 6.0	10.3 ± 6.0	10.5 ± 6.0		0.693

Notes: Results are presented as the means ± SDs or percentages. ED, emergency department, SD: standard deviation and CI: confidence interval.

In the bivariate analyses, only polypharmacy was associated with fall severity (OR: 1.63 [95% CI: 1.33–2.02]) (Table 1). The other clinical characteristics were not associated with fall severity. When the number of drugs was considered in categories with 0–3 drugs as the reference, we observed that the categories 4–6 (OR: 1.46 [1.00–2.14]) and 7–9 drugs (OR: 1.65 [1.09–2.50]) were associated with fall severity, whereas the category ≥10 drugs (N = 42 patients) (OR: 1.48 [0.76–2.85]) was not (Table 2). The percentages of fall severity were 38.1%, 47.3%, 50.3% and 47.6% for 0–3 drugs, 4–6 drugs, 7–9 drugs and ≥10 drugs, respectively (Table 2).

Table 2. Association between the number of drugs and need for hospital admission.

Number of Drugs	Percentage of Hospital Admission	Odds Ratio (95% CI)	*p*-Value
0–3 (n = 252)	38.1%	Reference	
4–6 (n = 188)	47.3%	1.46 [1.00–2.14]	0.049
7–9 (n = 143)	50.3%	1.65 [1.09–2.50]	0.018
≥10 (n = 42)	47.6%	1.48 [0.76–2.85]	0.244

CI, confidence interval.

4. Discussion

In this study, we observed that only polypharmacy (>5 drugs) was associated with hospital admission (OR: 1.63 [1.33–2.02]) in adults aged 70 years and over attending the ED of the University Hospital of Guadeloupe for a fall. This finding is consistent with a previous study by Morin et al. on a cohort of almost 50,000 patients, showing that there was an association between the number of medications prescribed and the risk of injurious falls [28]. In Morin's study, polypharmacy was defined as the use of than four medications (number of medications taken in the last 7 days and sorted according to the Anatomical Therapeutic Chemical (ATC) classification). The authors showed a 2% increase in falls among people taking multiple medications. However, after comprehensive adjustment for known confounders (including fall risk-increasing drugs and chronic multimorbidity), this association was substantially weaker than previously reported. Moreover, even if the relationship between polypharmacy and injurious falls is really causal, the population attributable risk fraction is low [28]. A similar association was also found by Laflamme et al. in a case–control study [29]. They found an increased risk of fall injury after two treatments [29].

In our study, when categorizing the number of medications taken, using the group taking 0–3 drugs as the reference category, we observed an increased risk of fall severity among older adults taking 4–6 medications and 7–9 medications. Nevertheless, no association was observed in the case of excessive polypharmacy (≥10 drugs), contrary to the studies by Laflamme et al. and Morin et al., where the relationship persisted at high numbers of drugs [28,29]. This difference compared to our work may be related to the difference in the main assessment criteria (i.e., definitions of fall severity and polypharmacy), as well as the sample size. The relatively small number of overmedicated patients (N = 42) in our study may contribute to the discrepancy between our findings and those reported in the existing literature. Indeed, we observed a similar rate of hospital admission in this subgroup (47.6%) compared to the 4–6 (47.3%) and 7–9 (50.3%) subgroup categories.

Further investigation is required to confirm these results. In this context, the administration of multiple drugs may be associated with therapeutic optimization strategies (in considering the quantitative and qualitative aspects of drugs) in this population, which are characterized by a high prevalence of underlying chronic pathologies. Patients with chronic conditions require a sufficient number of drugs to achieve therapeutic efficiency. Nevertheless, it is important to note that the risk of potential adverse health events remains high in patients receiving unnecessary treatments. It is therefore of the utmost importance that caution is exercised and that prescriptions are regularly reevaluated.

In our study, we did not find any association between cognitive impairment and fall severity. This finding is not consistent with the data in the literature, where it is well established that cognitive impairment is a risk factor for falls [24,30,31]. This lack of association may be partly due to the lack of power of the study or the lack of a precise diagnosis regarding cognitive impairment. Indeed, the data were retrieved from the patients' medical records, and no cognitive testing was performed during the ED visits. It is important to note that the majority of studies use the occurrence of a fracture (especially fractures of the upper end of the femur) as a criterion to assess the severity of a fall. After this type of fracture, the 6-month mortality rate for patients with a Mini Mental State Examination (MMSE) score < 20 is estimated to be 50%, compared to 11% for those with a normal MMSE score [32]. The threshold used by Tinetti was a MMSE < 26 (OR: 2.8 [95% CI: 1.7–4.7]) [33]. A history of repeated falls (≥2 falls in the previous 12 months) was not significantly associated with fall severity in our study. Repeated falls are predictive of adverse health events according to the French National Health Agency. However, 95% of recurrent falls are classified as non-serious, i.e., without fracture, cranial trauma or major skin laceration [5]. Several studies have shown that recurrent falls (>2 per year) are predictive of adverse health events in older people. These include incident dependency, hospitalization and mortality. This means that recurrent falls can be considered as a prognostic marker and/or a marker of fall severity (depending on the definition). The definition of fall severity (hospitalization and non-trauma) and the small number of patients in our study may explain the lack of significance. It should also be noted that the measurement of the "fall" variable may have lacked precision. Indeed, the local informatics database software does not include "history of falls" as a variable to be recorded during the clinical examination of older people. This information was only provided verbally during history taking or by reviewing the history of visits due to falls. Acute or chronic alcohol consumption also did not appear to be associated with fall severity in our study, but this may be due to the small number of persons in this category. Alcohol use is well known to be a risk factor for falls [34,35].

To the best of our knowledge, our study is the first to address the problem of falls among older adults in Guadeloupe. From a clinical point of view, our study highlights the value of optimizing medical therapy and thus fall prevention in older people. Our findings may contribute, albeit modestly, to changing current practices and to raising awareness about the impact of medication on the severity of falls. It may also form the basis for more in-depth future studies. In addition to international studies, our findings will encourage practitioners to minimize prescriptions as much as possible in older people (qualitative reduction or the concept of therapeutic optimization). Some limitations of our study should be noted. Firstly, patients were selected using the search engine integrated into the "statistics" function of the database software. It is plausible that some patients with falls may not have been identified by this search function and that the final number retained is not fully representative of all patients with falls aged 70 years and over who had an emergency department visit during this period. Second, this was a retrospective study. Third, medical records in the ED are completed for information purposes and mostly verbally, leading to a potential loss of information. Finally, the University Hospital of Guadeloupe experienced a period of crisis following an accidental fire at the facility in November 2017. The number of inpatient beds was drastically reduced (by around 200 beds), and this may have impacted the outcomes of patients who suffered falls because of a lack of downstream beds.

5. Conclusions

Our study showed an association between only polymedication (no link was identified between excessive polymedication) and fall severity in patients aged 70 years and over-attending the emergency department in Guadeloupe. This result highlights the cooccurrence of these two geriatric syndromes, which are most often managed by the attending physician. Longitudinal studies with larger numbers of patients are needed to explore the relationship between excessive polymedication and fall severity.

Author Contributions: N.S.-T. and M.T.T. designed the study and wrote the manuscript. G.M. contributed the data collection of patients' records. L.L., L.M., D.B.-M., L.R., L.V., M.-J.N.-E. and M.T.T. provided substantial feedback on the manuscript. All authors have read and agreed to the published version of the manuscript.

Funding: This research received no external funding.

Institutional Review Board Statement: The study protocol was approved by the Ethics Committee of the University Hospital of Guadeloupe on 25 August 2019, No. A7_19_08_09_CPPURG70.

Informed Consent Statement: Informed consent was obtained from all subjects involved in the study.

Data Availability Statement: All data generated or analyzed during this study are included in this published article. The datasets used and/or analyzed during the current study are available from the author Nadine Simo-Tabue upon reasonable request. The datasets generated and/or analyzed during the current study are not publicly available. The authors confirm that all experiments were performed in accordance with the relevant guidelines and regulations.

Conflicts of Interest: The authors declare that no conflicts of interest.

eferences

Tinetti, M.E.; Williams, C.S. The Effect of Falls and Fall Injuries on Functioning in Community-Dwelling Older Persons. *J. Gerontol. A. Biol. Sci. Med. Sci.* **1998**, *53*, M112–M119. [CrossRef]

Lewis, S.R.; McGarrigle, L.; Pritchard, M.W.; Bosco, A.; Yang, Y.; Gluchowski, A.; Sremanakova, J.; Boulton, E.R.; Gittins, M.; Spinks, A.; et al. Population-Based Interventions for Preventing Falls and Fall-Related Injuries in Older People. *Cochrane Database Syst. Rev.* **2024**, *1*, CD013789. [CrossRef]

Morris, M.E.; Webster, K.; Jones, C.; Hill, A.-M.; Haines, T.; McPhail, S.; Kiegaldie, D.; Slade, S.; Jazayeri, D.; Heng, H.; et al. Interventions to Reduce Falls in Hospitals: A Systematic Review and Meta-Analysis. *Age Ageing* **2022**, *51*, afac077. [CrossRef]

Xu, Q.; Ou, X.; Li, J. The Risk of Falls among the Aging Population: A Systematic Review and Meta-Analysis. *Front. Public Health* **2022**, *10*, 902599. [CrossRef]

Recommandations de La SFMU/Société Française de Médecine d'Urgence—SFMU. Available online: https://www.sfmu.org/fr/publications/recommandations-de-la-sfmu/evaluation-et-prise-en-charge-des-personnes-agees-faisant-des-chutes-repetees-/con_id/337 (accessed on 22 June 2024).

Schoene, D.; Heller, C.; Aung, Y.N.; Sieber, C.C.; Kemmler, W.; Freiberger, E. A Systematic Review on the Influence of Fear of Falling on Quality of Life in Older People: Is There a Role for Falls? *Clin. Interv. Aging* **2019**, *14*, 701–719. [CrossRef]

Durgun, H.; Turan, N.; Kaya, H. Relationship between Fall Behavior and Quality of Life of Elderly Individuals. *Psychol. Health Med.* **2022**, *27*, 1366–1372. [CrossRef]

Song, J.; Lee, E. Health-Related Quality of Life of Elderly Women with Fall Experiences. *Int. J. Environ. Res. Public Health* **2021**, *18*, 7804. [CrossRef] [PubMed]

Heinrich, S.; Rapp, K.; Rissmann, U.; Becker, C.; König, H.-H. Cost of Falls in Old Age: A Systematic Review. *Osteoporos. Int. J. Establ. Result Coop. Eur. Found. Osteoporos. Natl. Osteoporos. Found. USA* **2010**, *21*, 891–902. [CrossRef]

0. Montero-Odasso, M.M.; Kamkar, N.; Pieruccini-Faria, F.; Osman, A.; Sarquis-Adamson, Y.; Close, J.; Hogan, D.B.; Hunter, S.W.; Kenny, R.A.; Lipsitz, L.A.; et al. Evaluation of Clinical Practice Guidelines on Fall Prevention and Management for Older Adults: A Systematic Review. *JAMA Netw. Open* **2021**, *4*, e2138911. [CrossRef]

11. Phelan, E.A.; Ritchey, K. Fall Prevention in Community-Dwelling Older Adults. *Ann. Intern. Med.* **2018**, *169*, ITC81–ITC [CrossRef] [PubMed]
12. Gulka, H.J.; Patel, V.; Arora, T.; McArthur, C.; Iaboni, A. Efficacy and Generalizability of Falls Prevention Interventions in Nursi Homes: A Systematic Review and Meta-Analysis. *J. Am. Med. Dir. Assoc.* **2020**, *21*, 1024–1035.e4. [CrossRef]
13. Schultz, M.; Rosted, E.; Sanders, S. Frailty Is Associated with a History with More Falls in Elderly Hospitalised Patients. *D. Med. J.* **2015**, *62*, A5058.
14. Bischoff-Ferrari, H.A.; Freystätter, G.; Vellas, B.; Dawson-Hughes, B.; Kressig, R.W.; Kanis, J.A.; Willett, W.C.; Manson, J.E.; Rizz R.; Theiler, R.; et al. Effects of Vitamin D, Omega-3 Fatty Acids, and a Simple Home Strength Exercise Program on Fall Preventi The DO-HEALTH Randomized Clinical Trial. *Am. J. Clin. Nutr.* **2022**, *115*, 1311–1321. [CrossRef]
15. Guirguis-Blake, J.M.; Michael, Y.L.; Perdue, L.A.; Coppola, E.L.; Beil, T.L. Interventions to Prevent Falls in Older Adults: Updat Evidence Report and Systematic Review for the US Preventive Services Task Force. *JAMA* **2018**, *319*, 1705–1716. [CrossRef]
16. Wapp, C.; Biver, E.; Ferrari, S.; Zysset, P.; Zwahlen, M. Development of a Personalized Fall Rate Prediction Model in Communi Dwelling Older Adults: A Negative Binomial Regression Modelling Approach. *BMC Geriatr.* **2023**, *23*, 200. [CrossRef]
17. Le Floch, M.; Gautier, J.; Annweiler, C. Vitamin D Concentration and Motoric Cognitive Risk in Older Adults: Results from t Gait and Alzheimer Interactions Tracking (GAIT) Cohort. *Int. J. Environ. Res. Public Health* **2022**, *19*, 13086. [CrossRef]
18. Sampaio, F.; Nogueira, P.; Ascenção, R.; Henriques, A.; Costa, A. The Epidemiology of Falls in Portugal: An Analysis of Hospi Admission Data. *PLoS ONE* **2021**, *16*, e0261456. [CrossRef]
19. Vu, H.M.; Nguyen, L.H.; Nguyen, H.L.T.; Vu, G.T.; Nguyen, C.T.; Hoang, T.N.; Tran, T.H.; Pham, K.T.H.; Latkin, C.A.; Xuan Tra B.; et al. Individual and Environmental Factors Associated with Recurrent Falls in Elderly Patients Hospitalized after Falls. *Int. Environ. Res. Public Health* **2020**, *17*, 2441. [CrossRef]
20. Yoshida, Y.; Ishizaki, T.; Masui, Y.; Hori, N.; Inagaki, H.; Ito, K.; Ogawa, M.; Yasumoto, S.; Arai, Y.; Kamide, K.; et al. Effect Number of Medications on the Risk of Falls among Community-Dwelling Older Adults: A 3-Year Follow-up of the SONIC Stu *Geriatr. Gerontol. Int.* **2024**, *24*, 306–310. [CrossRef]
21. Masnoon, N.; Shakib, S.; Kalisch-Ellett, L.; Caughey, G.E. What Is Polypharmacy? A Systematic Review of Definitions. *BM Geriatr.* **2017**, *17*, 230. [CrossRef]
22. Pazan, F.; Wehling, M. Polypharmacy in Older Adults: A Narrative Review of Definitions, Epidemiology and Consequences. *E Geriatr. Med.* **2021**, *12*, 443–452. [CrossRef] [PubMed]
23. Delara, M.; Murray, L.; Jafari, B.; Bahji, A.; Goodarzi, Z.; Kirkham, J.; Chowdhury, M.; Seitz, D.P. Prevalence and Facto Associated with Polypharmacy: A Systematic Review and Meta-Analysis. *BMC Geriatr.* **2022**, *22*, 601. [CrossRef]
24. James, K.; Eldemire-Shearer, D.; Gouldbourne, J.; Morris, C. Falls and Fall Prevention in the Elderly. *West Indian Med. J.* **2007**, 5 534. [PubMed]
25. Lyons, B.P.; Hall, R.J. Outcomes of a Falls Prevention Education Program Among Older Adults in Grenada. *J. Community Healt* **2016**, *41*, 1021–1026. [CrossRef]
26. Yogi, R.R.; Sammy, I.; Paul, J.F.; Nunes, P.; Robertson, P.; Ramcharitar Maharaj, V. Falls in Older People: Comparing Older an Younger Fallers in a Developing Country. *Eur. J. Trauma Emerg. Surg. Off. Publ. Eur. Trauma Soc.* **2018**, *44*, 567–571. [CrossRef]
27. Welter, M.-L.; Vasseur, A.; Edragas, R.; Chaumont, H.; Pineau, F.; Mangone, G.; Olivier, C.; Leber, I.; Rivaud-Pechoux, S.; Leheric S.; et al. Brain Dysfunction in Gait Disorders of Caribbean Atypical Parkinsonism and Progressive Supranuclear Palsy Patients: Comparative Study. *NeuroImage Clin.* **2023**, *38*, 103443. [CrossRef] [PubMed]
28. Morin, L.; Calderon Larrañaga, A.; Welmer, A.-K.; Rizzuto, D.; Wastesson, J.W.; Johnell, K. Polypharmacy and Injurious Falls i Older Adults: A Nationwide Nested Case-Control Study. *Clin. Epidemiol.* **2019**, *11*, 483–493. [CrossRef]
29. Laflamme, L.; Monárrez-Espino, J.; Johnell, K.; Elling, B.; Möller, J. Type, Number or Both? A Population-Based Matche Case-Control Study on the Risk of Fall Injuries among Older People and Number of Medications beyond Fall-Inducing Drugs *PLoS ONE* **2015**, *10*, e0123390. [CrossRef]
30. Ensrud, K.E.; Ewing, S.K.; Cawthon, P.M.; Fink, H.A.; Taylor, B.C.; Cauley, J.A.; Dam, T.-T.; Marshall, L.M.; Orwoll, E.S. Cummings, S.R.; et al. A Comparison of Frailty Indexes for the Prediction of Falls, Disability, Fractures, and Mortality in Olde Men. *J. Am. Geriatr. Soc.* **2009**, *57*, 492–498. [CrossRef]
31. Strubel, D.; Jacquot, J.M.; Martin-Hunyadi, C. [Dementia and falls]. *Ann. Readaptation Med. Phys. Rev. Sci. Soc. Francais Reeducation Fonct. Readaptation Med. Phys.* **2001**, *44*, 4–12. [CrossRef]
32. Lyons, A.R. Clinical Outcomes and Treatment of Hip Fractures. *Am. J. Med.* **1997**, *103*, 51S–63S, discussion 63S–64S. [CrossRef] [PubMed]
33. Tinetti, M.E.; Doucette, J.T.; Claus, E.B. The Contribution of Predisposing and Situational Risk Factors to Serious Fall Injuries. *J Am. Geriatr. Soc.* **1995**, *43*, 1207–1213. [CrossRef] [PubMed]

Zautcke, J.L.; Coker, S.B.; Morris, R.W.; Stein-Spencer, L. Geriatric Trauma in the State of Illinois: Substance Use and Injury Patterns. *Am. J. Emerg. Med.* **2002**, *20*, 14–17. [CrossRef] [PubMed]
Stenbacka, M.; Jansson, B.; Leifman, A.; Romelsjö, A. Association between Use of Sedatives or Hypnotics, Alcohol Consumption, or Other Risk Factors and a Single Injurious Fall or Multiple Injurious Falls: A Longitudinal General Population Study. *Alcohol* **2002**, *28*, 9–16. [CrossRef] [PubMed]

healthcare

MDPI

Article

Predictive Validity of the Johns Hopkins Fall Risk Assessment Tool for Older Patients in Stroke Rehabilitation

Seungho Hong [1], Ji-Sook Kim [2] and Young-Ah Choi [1,*]

[1] Department of Rehabilitation Medicine, Incheon St. Mary's Hospital, College of Medicine, The Catholic University of Korea, Seoul 06591, Republic of Korea

[2] Department of Nursing, Incheon St. Mary's Hospital, The Catholic University of Korea, Incheon 21431, Republic of Korea

* Correspondence: simple16@catholic.ac.kr; Tel.: +82-032-280-6601

Abstract: The aim of this retrospective, cross-sectional, observational study was to assess the frequency of falls and evaluate the predictive validity of the Johns Hopkins Fall Risk Assessment Tool (JHFRAT) among patients aged ≥65 years, transferred to the rehabilitation ward of a university hospital. The predictive ability was assessed using receiver operating characteristic curve analysis, and the optimal threshold was established using the Youden index. We analyzed the overall cohort (N = 175) with subacute stroke and the subgroup with a low unaffected handgrip strength (HGS; men: <28 kg, women: <18 kg). Overall, 135/175 patients (77.1%) had a low HGS. The fall rate was 6.9% overall and 5.9% for patients with a low HGS. The JHFRAT predictive value was higher for patients with a low HGS than that for the overall cohort, but acceptable in both. The optimal cutoff score for the overall cohort was 11 (sensitivity, 67%; specificity, 68%), whereas that for the subgroup was 12 (sensitivity, 75%; specificity: 72%). These results are expected to aid nurses working in rehabilitation wards in more effectively utilizing JHFRAT outcomes for post-stroke older patients with a low HGS and contribute to the development of more appropriate fall prevention strategies for high-risk patients in the future.

Keywords: fall; stroke; rehabilitation; handgrip strength

1. Introduction

A fall can be defined as "an event which results in a person coming to rest inadvertently on the ground or floor or other lower level" [1], although the definition of a fall is not standardized [2]. With the aging of the population worldwide, falls are a substantial public health concern because of the potential for unexpected injuries [3,4]. Falls are associated with fractures, serious soft tissue injuries requiring medical attention, increased dependence for daily activities, and fear of falling among people aged 65 years and older [5]. Especially for hospitalized older patients, falls can be fatal as they can worsen the underlying disease and lead to new injuries, impairing the patient's recovery [6,7].

Falls have various causes in older people, most notably decreased musculoskeletal function [5], such as muscle weakness. Prior research has consistently revealed a heightened likelihood of falls by individuals presenting with a diminished handgrip strength (HGS) [8–11]. For instance, in a longitudinal study conducted among residents of mainland China aged 45 years and older, weak grip strength was reported as a risk factor for falls [8]. Similarly, in a prospective study involving community-dwelling women, reduced grip strength was independently associated with a higher risk of falls in older women [9]. A meta-analysis revealed that decreased upper-extremity strength was associated with a 53% increased risk of falls [10]. These findings underscore the potential utility of HGS in predicting fall risk and in stratification in both clinical and research contexts.

Consequently, fall prevention has emerged as a crucial aspect of geriatric care, particularly after an acute stroke. The prompt initiation of rehabilitation, ideally within a few days of the onset of stroke symptoms, is crucial, as early mobilization is closely related to better functional outcomes at discharge and a shorter hospital stay [12]. However, fall-related injuries substantially hinder the rehabilitation process. Therefore, efforts to identify the risk factors for falls, such as the development of risk assessment tools, are ongoing [13]. For example, Joint Commission International (JCI), a nonprofit organization that certifies the quality of patient safety in healthcare organizations, requires fall risk assessment and prevention practices for healthcare institute accreditation because falls lead to longer hospital stays, increased medical costs, and even death [14].

The Johns Hopkins Fall Risk Assessment Tool (JHFRAT) is widely used to prevent falls. Compared to other fall risk assessment tools, it is efficient in assessing fall risk and managing high-risk groups upon hospitalization [15], and the JHFRAT has been validated in various acute care departments across different acute care units [16]. As the JHFRAT is easy to implement, repeated assessments can be used to monitor changes in a patient's condition. In a study on the reliability and predictive validity of the JHFRAT, the total JHFRAT score had an acceptable inter-rater agreement among four types of acute care units, as well as high sensitivity [16]. According to JCI, the provision of more intensive fall prevention programs necessitates the initial use of tools capable of appropriately assessing fall risk, allowing for the development of suitable systems within each care setting. Studies in Korea [17] and China [15] in which the validity of the JHFRAT was evaluated among the acutely hospitalized general population encompassing all adult age groups suggested that it is a reliable fall risk assessment tool in acute inpatient settings. However, the statistical characteristics of the JHFRAT are reportedly inconsistent, such as its predictive validity. For instance, its sensitivity and specificity vary across studies; in some studies, it has a low sensitivity but high specificity, and in other studies, it has a higher specificity than sensitivity [16]. This discrepancy underscores the need to apply fall risk assessment tools in a customized manner to accurately evaluate the potential for falls during hospitalization owing to the variability of patient conditions in acute care environments.

Stroke is an additional risk factor for falls, especially among older patients [18,19], owing to stroke-related motor, sensory, and visual deficits, which impair balance and reduce functional mobility [20]. The incidence of falls in patients with acute stroke ranges from 8.7% to 39% [3,21,22]. In acute-stroke units, patient activity is typically restricted to bed rest. However, in rehabilitation wards, mobility is increased, which leads to a higher incidence of falls. Furthermore, in university hospitals, a large proportion of patients in the stroke rehabilitation wards are older individuals. However, fall risk assessment tools specifically designed for older patients with stroke have not been standardized. Furthermore, the predictive ability of JHFRAT among older patients with stroke is unclear.

The aim of this study was to assess the frequency of falls and the utility of the JHFRAT among older patients with stroke who had been transferred to the rehabilitation ward of a university hospital. Furthermore, considering that reduced HGS is a significant risk factor for falls in older adults [9,10] and is closely related to frailty [23], we evaluated the predictive validity of the JHFRAT not only among all stroke patients aged ≥65 years admitted to the rehabilitation ward but also specifically among those with a decreased HGS on the unaffected side. We hypothesized that tailored application of the JHFRAT to assess the fall risk in older patients during the subacute phase of stroke rehabilitation not only extends the tool's utility beyond general acute care but also improves diagnostic accuracy. We believe that such customization of fall risk assessment tools for specialized acute care settings will enhance the effectiveness of fall prevention strategies.

2. Materials and Methods

2.1. Study Population

This retrospective study included patients who were diagnosed with acute cerebral infarction or hemorrhage and transferred to the rehabilitation ward from March 2021 to June 2023 at a tertiary university hospital. Inclusion criteria were as follows: (1) age ≥65 years, (2) diagnosed with acute stroke using magnetic resonance imaging or computed tomography, and (3) evaluated with the JHFRAT at the time of transfer to the rehabilitation ward. The exclusion criteria were as follows: (1) JHFRAT assessment not conducted at the time of transfer to the rehabilitation ward, and (2) an inability to complete the initial functional assessment, including that for HGS, due to circumstances such as premature discharge or medical issues. This study was approved by the institutional review board (IRB) of the tertiary hospital, and all methods were performed in accordance with the Code of Ethics of the World Medical Association (Declaration of Helsinki). Owing to the retrospective nature of the study, patient consent was waived by the IRB.

2.2. JHFRAT

The JHFRAT is a mandatory screening tool for JCI certification and is used at the university hospital where the study was conducted. The Korean version of the JHFRAT is administered within 24 h of admission and weekly thereafter [17]. The JHFRAT scores obtained during the week of transfer to the rehabilitation ward were collected for analysis. The JHFRAT first differentiates between direct high- and low-risk groups based on a patient's fall history and mobility. If a patient was assigned to either category, the risk score was not measured. In most previous studies, the direct high-risk group was not identified or they were not excluded from the analysis [16,24]. In our study, none of the patients could be assigned to the direct high- or low-risk groups. Therefore, all patients who underwent the JHFRAT measurement in our study population were included in this study. The fall risk score is based on age at admission, 6-month fall history before admission, elimination of the bowel and bladder, use of medications (such as sedatives and antihypertensive drugs) that pose a high fall risk, the presence of patient care equipment that tethers the patient, mobility problems, and cognitive dysfunction. The JHFRAT score ranges from 0 to 35 points, and scores of <6, 6–13, and >13 were classified as low, moderate, and high fall risk, respectively. As only individuals aged ≥65 years were included, the lowest score for the age item was 1. Furthermore, because the mobility and cognition items involved the selection of multiple options, they were presented as continuous variables. The remaining items were all single-option items and were, thus, categorized as categorical variables.

2.3. Monitoring of Falls

Fall monitoring is accomplished through the continuous and systematic observation of hospitalized patients. If a patient falls during their hospital stay, a nurse records it in the system for reporting adverse events and enters it into the patient's electronic health record. Physicians reviewed the participants' medical records to retrospectively verify each fall by assessing the circumstances reported for the fall.

2.4. Measurement of HGS

The HGS of the unaffected side was measured by a trained occupational therapist at the time of transfer to the rehabilitation ward. The measurement was performed three times using a Jamar dynamometer (Lafayette, IN, USA), and the highest value was used for the analysis. According to the sarcopenia diagnosis algorithm of the Asian Working Group for Sarcopenia, an HGS of <28 kg in men and <18 kg in women was considered indicative of a low HGS [25].

2.5. Data Collection

Demographic data and clinical variables related to the fall risk were collected via retrospective chart review [5,22,26,27]. These included age, sex, body mass index, history of stroke, days since stroke onset, stroke lesion type (ischemic vs. hemorrhagic), stroke severity according to the National Institutes of Health Stroke Scale, and total length of stay. Regarding the functional impairment after stroke, the patient's balancing function was quantitatively assessed using the Berg Balance Scale, and the motor function of the hemiplegic lower extremity was assessed using the Fugl–Meyer assessment. The activities of daily living were evaluated using the Korean version of the modified Barthel Index. Cognitive function was assessed using the Korean version of the mini-mental state examination-2, and depression was assessed using the Beck Depression Inventory. Furthermore, clinical variables that contributed to the fall risk due to stroke were investigated, except for those that overlapped with the JHFRAT items. These were aphasia, spatial neglect, visual field and visual acuity problems, hearing loss, and the total number of medications used.

2.6. Statistical Analysis

Data for continuous variables that followed a normal distribution are indicated as the mean and standard deviation, and those that were not normally distributed are presented as the median [interquartile range]. We assessed the data distribution of each variable using the Kolmogorov–Smirnov test to confirm normality. Categorical variables are presented as frequencies and percentages. We explored potential discrepancies in clinical variables between the groups by applying Student's *t*-test or the Mann–Whitney *U* test for continuous variables, and Pearson's chi-square test or Fisher's exact test for categorical variables. The overall predictive ability of the JHFRAT was evaluated using the area under the receiver operating characteristic (ROC) curve (AUC), and the optimal cutoff point was calculated for the entire sample as well as for the group with a low HGS, according to the value with the highest Youden index [28]. All statistical analyses were performed using R software (R-4.3.1). Statistical significance was set at $p < 0.05$.

3. Results

Of the 210 patients diagnosed with acute stroke during the study period, 175 patients (71 men and 104 women) aged ≥65 years were finally included for analysis. Among these 175 patients, 135 (77.1%) had a low HGS on the non-hemiplegic side. The median age of the sample was 76 [70.0–82.0] years, and the proportion of men was 40.6% (n = 71). The median age of the group with a low HGS was 78 [72.0–83.0] years, and the proportion of men was 38.5% (n = 52). The baseline characteristics of the overall sample and those of patients with a low HGS are summarized in Table 1. The fall rate from transfer to the neurorehabilitation ward until discharge was 6.9% (12 of 175) in the entire cohort. Among patients with a low HGS, the fall rate was 5.9% (8 of 135). None of the patients had experienced falls before admission or before transfer to the rehabilitation ward.

Table 1. Baseline characteristics of all patients and those with a low HGS.

Variables	All Patients (N = 175)	Patients with Low HGS (n = 135)
Age, years	76.0 [70.0–82.0]	78.0 [72.0–83.0]
Sex		
Male	71 (40.6%)	52 (38.5%)
Female	104 (59.4%)	83 (61.5%)
BMI, kg/m^2	23.5 [21.4–26.8]	23.4 [20.9–26.8]
Stroke history		
First	128 (73.1%)	94 (69.6%)
Recurrent (2nd)	34 (19.4%)	29 (21.5%)
Recurrent (3rd)	13 (7.4%)	12 (8.9%)
Time from onset of stroke to transfer, days	12.0 [8.0–17.0]	14.0 [8.0–18.5]
Lesion		
Ischemic	146 (83.4%)	109 (80.7%)
Hemorrhagic	29 (16.6%)	26 (19.3%)
NIHSS score	4.0 [2.0–8.0]	4.0 [2.0–9.0]
LOS, days	41.0 [32.0–52.0]	42.0 [33.0–53.0]
HGS of non-hemiplegic hand, kg	14.0 [8.0–22.0]	11.0 [4.0–16.0]
BBS score	8.0 [2.0–29.0]	6.0 [1.0–22.0]
FMA score of hemiplegic lower extremity	24.0 [8.5–29.0]	22.0 [6.0–28.5]
MBI	24.0 [7.0–45.5]	13.0 [5.0–39.0]
MMSE score	17.0 [10.5–23.5]	15.0 [8.0–21.0]
BDI score	13.0 [7.0–25.0]	15.0 [7.0–26.0]

Table 1. *Cont.*

Variables	All Patients (N = 175)	Patients with Low HGS (n = 135)
Aphasia		
Absence	114 (65.1%)	82 (60.7%)
Presence	61 (34.9%)	53 (39.3%)
Spatial neglect		
Absence	159 (90.9%)	122 (90.4%)
Presence	16 (9.1%)	13 (9.6%)
Visual field problems		
Absence	168 (96.0%)	129 (95.6%)
Presence	7 (4.0%)	6 (4.4%)
Visual acuity problems		
Absence	168 (96.0%)	132 (97.8%)
Presence	7 (4.0%)	3 (2.2%)
Hearing loss		
Absence	162 (92.6%)	127 (94.1%)
Presence	13 (7.4%)	8 (5.9%)
Total number of medications used	10.2 ± 3.1	10.4 ± 3.1
Falls		
No	163 (93.1%)	127 (94.1%)
Yes	12 (6.9%)	8 (5.9%)

Data are expressed as the frequency (proportion), mean ± standard deviation, or median [interquartile range]. HGS, handgrip strength; BMI, body mass index; NIHSS, National Institutes of Health Stroke Scale; LOS, length of stay; BBS, Berg Balance Scale; FMA, Fugl–Meyer assessment; MBI, modified Barthel Index; MMSE, mini-mental state examination; BDI, Beck Depression Inventory.

Comparisons of patients who experienced falls and those who did not revealed no significant differences in age, sex, clinical variables, or functional outcomes among the overall cohort or among the group with a low HGS (Table 2). However, among those with a low HGS, patients who experienced falls had a longer median duration from stroke onset to transfer to the rehabilitation ward (20.5 [15.0–30.0] days) than their counterparts who did not experience falls (13.0 [8.0–18.0] days).

The scores for each JHFRAT item and the overall JHFRAT score were compared according to whether falls occurred, both in the entire cohort and in the low-HGS group, and the distribution of patients who experienced falls and those who did not is presented in Figure 1 according to the JHFRAT score. In the study sample, the minimum score was 1, the median score was 8, and the maximum score was 21. In the group with a low HGS, the minimum and maximum scores were the same, and the median score was 9.

Upon ROC curve analysis, the AUC was 0.67 (95% confidence interval [CI]: 0.49–0.67) for the overall cohort and 0.74 (95% CI: 0.54–0.74) for patients with a low HGS (Figure 2). For the group with a lower HGS, the AUC was higher than that for the overall cohort. For both groups, the sensitivity, specificity, positive predictive value (PPV), and negative predictive value (NPV) of the JHFRAT were further assessed using the Youden index (Table 3). Among the overall cohort, the JHFRAT cutoff score yielding the maximal Youden index (0.35) was 11, and the sensitivity, specificity, PPV, and NPV at that score were 0.67, 0.68, 13%, and 97%, respectively. Among patients with a low HGS, the cutoff score yielding the maximal Youden index (0.47) was 12, and the sensitivity, specificity, PPV, and NPV at that score were 0.75, 0.72, 14%, and 98%, respectively.

Table 2. Baseline characteristics of patients classified according to HGS and falls.

Variable	All Patients				Patients with Low HGS			
	Non-Fallers (n = 163)	Fallers (n = 12)	Total (N = 175)	*p*	Non-Fallers (n = 127)	Fallers (n = 8)	Total (N = 135)	*p*
Age, years	76.0 [70.0–82.0]	79.0 [72.0–81.5]	76.0 [70.0–82.0]	0.552	77.0 [72.0–83.0]	79.5 [78.0–82.0]	78.0 [72.0–83.0]	0.508
Sex				0.701				>0.999
Male	65 (39.9%)	6 (50.0%)	71 (40.6%)		49 (38.6%)	3 (37.5%)	52 (38.5%)	
Female	98 (60.1%)	6 (50.0%)	104 (59.4%)		78 (61.4%)	5 (62.5%)	83 (61.5%)	
BMI, kg/m^2	23.5 [21.5–26.8]	22.8 [20.6–28.1]	23.5 [21.4–26.8]	0.969	23.5 [21.2–26.8]	21.3 [19.6–25.8]	23.4 [20.9–26.8]	0.278
Stroke history				0.557				0.657
First	119 (73.0%)	9 (75.0%)	128 (73.1%)		88 (69.3%)	6 (75.0%)	94 (69.6%)	
Recurrent (2nd)	31 (19.0%)	3 (25.0%)	34 (19.4%)		27 (21.3%)	2 (25.0%)	29 (21.5%)	
Recurrent (3rd)	13 (8.0%)	0 (0.0%)	13 (7.4%)		12 (9.4%)	0 (0.0%)	12 (8.9%)	
Time from onset of stroke to transfer, days	12.0 [8.0–17.0]	15.0 [9.0–24.5]	12.0 [8.0–17.0]	0.252	13.0 [8.0–18.0]	20.5 [15.0–30.0]	14.0 [8.0–18.5]	0.030 *
Lesion				0.681				0.375
Ischemic	137 (84.0%)	9 (75.0%)	146 (83.4%)		104 (81.9%)	5 (62.5%)	109 (80.7%)	
Hemorrhagic	26 (16.0%)	3 (25.0%)	29 (16.6%)		23 (18.1%)	3 (37.5%)	26 (19.3%)	
NIHSS score	4.0 [2.0–8.0]	4.5 [0.5–5.0]	4.0 [2.0–8.0]	0.248	4.0 [2.0–9.0]	3.5 [0.5–7.0]	4.0 [2.0–9.0]	0.230
LOS, days	40.0 [32.0–51.5]	45.5 [34.0–52.0]	41.0 [32.0–52.0]	0.425	42.0 [33.0–53.0]	48.5 [34.5–57.0]	42.0 [33.0–53.0]	0.439
HGS of non-hemiplegic hand, kg	14.0 [6.8–20.0]	20.0 [10.0–27.0]	14.0 [8.0–22.0]	0.171	11.0 [4.0–16.0]	11.0 [9.0–20.0]	11.0 [4.0–16.0]	0.559
BBS score	7.0 [2.0–28.5]	16.0 [7.0–47.5]	8.0 [2.0–29.0]	0.061	6.0 [1.0–22.0]	11.0 [6.5–33.0]	6.0 [1.0–22.0]	0.237
FMA score of hemiplegic lower extremity	22.0 [8.0–29.0]	26.5 [24.0–30.5]	24.0 [8.5–29.0]	0.090	21.0 [6.0–28.0]	26.5 [24.0–31.5]	22.0 [6.0–28.5]	0.087
MBI	22.0 [6.5–45.5]	37.0 [16.5–56.0]	24.0 [7.0–45.5]	0.212	13.0 [4.5–39.0]	28.5 [10.0–56.0]	13.0 [5.0–39.0]	0.277
MMSE score	17.0 [10.0–23.0]	21.0 [12.5–27.5]	17.0 [10.5–23.5]	0.242	15.0 [8.0–21.0]	14.5 [9.0–21.5]	15.0 [8.0–21.0]	0.948
BDI score	13.0 [7.0–25.0]	12.0 [6.5–24.0]	13.0 [7.0–25.0]	0.887	15.0 [7.0–26.0]	14.0 [6.0–34.5]	15.0 [7.0–26.0]	0.830
Aphasia				>0.999				>0.999
Absence	106 (65.0%)	8 (66.7%)	114 (65.1%)		77 (60.6%)	5 (62.5%)	82 (60.7%)	
Presence	57 (35.0%)	4 (33.3%)	61 (34.9%)		50 (39.4%)	3 (37.5%)	53 (39.3%)	
Spatial neglect				0.535				0.738
Absence	147 (90.2%)	12 (100.0%)	159 (90.9%)		114 (89.8%)	8 (100.0%)	122 (90.4%)	
Presence	16 (9.8%)	0 (0.0%)	16 (9.1%)		13 (10.2%)	0 (0.0%)	13 (9.6%)	
Visual field problems				>0.999				>0.999
Absence	156 (95.7%)	12 (100.0%)	168 (96.0%)		121 (95.3%)	8 (100.0%)	129 (95.6%)	
Presence	7 (4.3%)	0 (0.0%)	7 (4.0%)		6 (4.7%)	0 (0.0%)	6 (4.4%)	
Visual acuity problems				0.976				0.426
Absence	157 (96.3%)	11 (91.7%)	168 (96.0%)		125 (98.4%)	7 (87.5%)	132 (97.8%)	
Presence	6 (3.7%)	1 (8.3%)	7 (4.0%)		2 (1.6%)	1 (12.5%)	3 (2.2%)	
Hearing loss				>0.999				>0.999
Absence	151 (92.6%)	11 (91.7%)	162 (92.6%)		119 (93.7%)	8 (100.0%)	127 (94.1%)	
Presence	12 (7.4%)	1 (8.3%)	13 (7.4%)		8 (6.3%)	0 (0.0%)	8 (5.9%)	
Total number of medications used	10.2 ± 3.0	11.1 ± 4.5	10.2 ± 3.1	0.500	10.3 ± 3.0	11.6 ± 4.9	10.4 ± 3.1	0.474

Data are expressed as the frequency (proportion), mean ± standard deviation, or median [interquartile range]. HGS, handgrip strength; BMI, body mass index; NIHSS, National Institutes of Health Stroke Scale; LOS, length of stay; BBS, Berg Balance Scale; FMA, Fugl–Meyer assessment; MBI, modified Barthel Index; MMSE, mini-mental state examination; BDI, Beck Depression Inventory. Differences that are statistically significant are indicated with an asterisk, signifying $p < 0.05$.

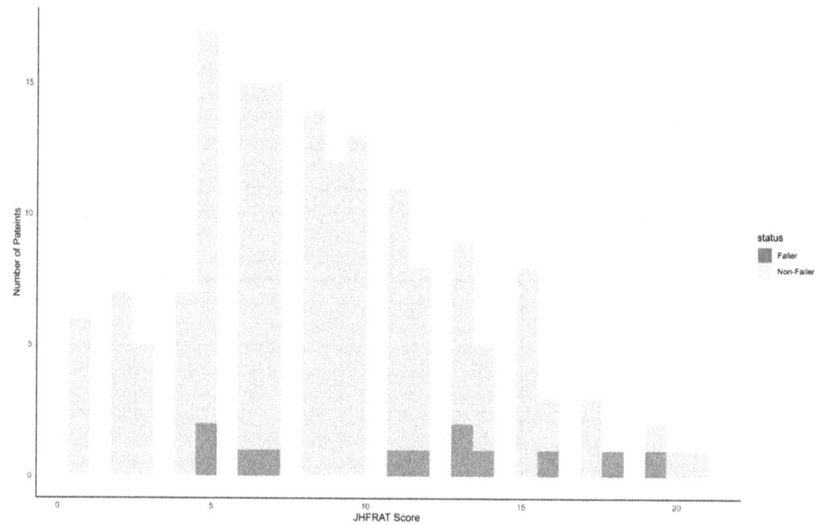

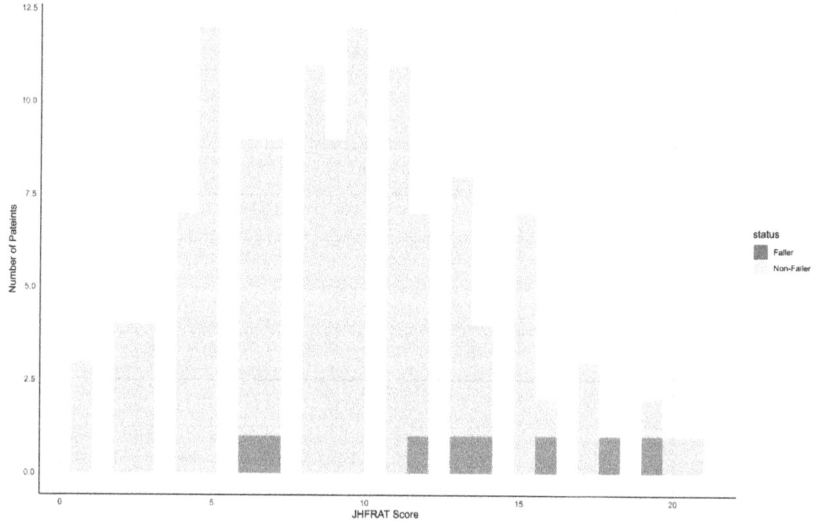

Figure 1. Number of patients who experienced falls and those who did not according to the JHFRAT score during their stay in the rehabilitation ward. Overall cohort (**upper**). Patients with a low HGS (**lower**). JHFRAT, Johns Hopkins Fall Risk Assessment Tool; HGS, handgrip strength.

In the entire study cohort, the proportion of patients with urgent, frequent, or incontinent problems in the "Intestinal and urinary elimination" category differed between those who had experienced falls and those who had not. However, no significant intergroup differences were observed in the other categories or in the total JHFRAT score in the overall cohort. In contrast, in the group with a low HGS, the proportion of patients using medication posing a high risk of falls was higher among those who had experienced falls, as was the prevalence of urgent, frequent, or incontinent problems in the "Intestinal and urinary elimination" category. Furthermore, in the low-HGS group, the average total JHFRAT score of patients who had not experienced falls and those who had was 9.2 ± 4.4 and 13.1 ± 4.7, respectively, indicating a significantly higher overall JHFRAT score among those who had experienced falls ($p = 0.016$; Table 4).

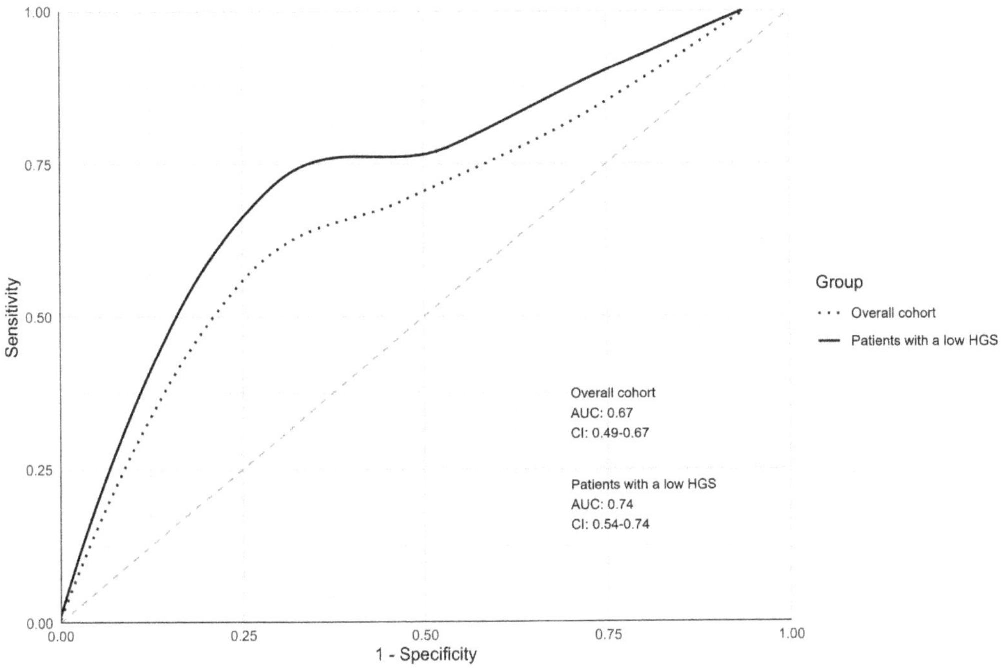

Figure 2. Comparison of the predictive efficacy of the Johns Hopkins Fall Risk Assessment Tool (JHFRAT) in the overall cohort and older adults with low HGS. AUC, area under the curve; CI, confidence interval; HGS, handgrip strength; ROC, receiver operating characteristic.

Table 3. Sensitivity, specificity, PPV, and NPV of the JHFRAT at different cutoff scores.

Group	Cutoff Score	Sensitivity	Specificity	PPV (95% CI)	NPV (95% CI)	Youden Index
Total cohort	6	0.83	0.26	0.08 (0.04–0.14)	0.95 (0.85–0.99)	0.09
	7	0.75	0.35	0.08 (0.04–0.14)	0.95 (0.86–0.99)	0.10
	8	0.67	0.44	0.08 (0.04–0.15)	0.95 (0.87–0.99)	0.11
	9	0.67	0.53	0.09 (0.04–0.18)	0.96 (0.89–0.99)	0.19
	10	0.67	0.60	0.11 (0.05–0.20)	0.96 (0.90–0.99)	0.27
	11	0.67	0.68	0.13 (0.06–0.25)	0.97 (0.91–0.99)	0.35
	12	0.58	0.75	0.15 (0.06–0.28)	0.96 (0.91–0.99)	0.33
	13	0.50	0.80	0.15 (0.06–0.31)	0.96 (0.91–0.98)	0.30
Patients with low HGS	6	1.00	0.24	0.08 (0.03–0.14)	1.00 (0.88–1.00)	0.24
	7	0.88	0.31	0.07 (0.03–0.15)	0.97 (0.87–1.00)	0.18
	8	0.75	0.38	0.07 (0.03–0.15)	0.96 (0.86–1.00)	0.13
	9	0.75	0.46	0.08 (0.03–0.17)	0.97 (0.89–1.00)	0.21
	10	0.75	0.54	0.09 (0.03–0.19)	0.97 (0.90–1.00)	0.29
	11	0.75	0.63	0.11 (0.04–0.23)	0.98 (0.91–1.00)	0.38
	12	0.75	0.72	0.14 (0.05–0.29)	0.98 (0.92–1.00)	0.47
	13	0.62	0.77	0.15 (0.05–0.31)	0.97 (0.92–0.99)	0.40

For both the overall cohort and the group of patients with a low HGS, the *p*-values for both positive and negative predictive values at each cutoff score were significant, being less than 0.001. PPV, positive predictive value; NPV, negative predictive value; JHFRAT, Johns Hopkins Fall Risk Assessment Tool; CI, confidence interval; HGS, handgrip strength.

Table 4. Adaptation of the Johns Hopkins Fall Risk Assessment Tool in older patients according to HGS and fall events.

	Total Cohort				Patients with Low HGS			
	Non-Fallers (n = 163)	**Fallers (n = 12)**	**Total (N = 175)**	***p***	**Non-Fallers (n = 127)**	**Fallers (n = 8)**	**Total (N = 135)**	***p***
Age (years)				0.462				0.779
60–69	40 (24.5%)	2 (16.7%)	42 (24.0%)		23 (18.1%)	1 (12.5%)	24 (17.8%)	
70–79	70 (42.9%)	4 (33.3%)	74 (42.3%)		56 (44.1%)	3 (37.5%)	59 (43.7%)	
≥80	53 (32.5%)	6 (50.0%)	59 (33.7%)		48 (37.8%)	4 (50.0%)	52 (38.5%)	
History of one fall within 6 months before admission				0.850				0.534
No	146 (89.6%)	10 (83.3%)	156 (89.1%)		113 (89.0%)	6 (75.0%)	119 (88.1%)	
Yes	17 (10.4%)	2 (16.7%)	19 (10.9%)		14 (11.0%)	2 (25.0%)	16 (11.9%)	
Intestinal and urinary elimination				0.002 *				0.033 *
Normal	157 (96.3%)	9 (75.0%)	166 (94.8%)		121 (95.3%)	6 (75.0%)	127 (94.1%)	
Incontinence or urgency or frequency	5 (3.1%)	3 (25.0%)	8 (4.6%)		5 (3.9%)	2 (25.0%)	7 (5.2%)	
Urgency/frequency and incontinence	1 (0.6%)	0 (0.0%)	1 (0.6%)		1 (0.8%)	0 (0.0%)	1 (0.7%)	
Use of drugs entailing high risk of falls				0.255				0.024 *
None	132 (81.0%)	8 (66.7%)	140 (80.0%)		103 (81.1%)	5 (62.5%)	108 (80.0%)	
1 high fall-risk drug	28 (17.2%)	3 (25.0%)	31 (17.7%)		23 (18.1%)	2 (25.0%)	25 (18.5%)	
2 or more high fall-risk drug	3 (1.8%)	1 (8.3%)	4 (2.3%)		1 (0.8%)	1 (12.5%)	2 (1.5%)	
Equipment that may compromise mobility				0.427				0.242
No	102 (62.6%)	7 (58.3%)	109 (62.3%)		73 (57.5%)	3 (37.5%)	76 (56.3%)	
1	34 (20.9%)	3 (25.0%)	37 (21.1%)		29 (22.8%)	3 (37.5%)	32 (23.7%)	
2	16 (9.8%)	0 (0.0%)	16 (9.1%)		14 (11.0%)	0 (0.0%)	14 (10.4%)	
≥3	11 (6.7%)	2 (16.7%)	13 (7.4%)		11 (8.7%)	2 (25.0%)	13 (9.6%)	
Mobility impairment	2.4 ± 1.6	3.2 ± 1.3	2.5 ± 1.6	0.121	2.3 ± 1.5	3.0 ± 1.5	2.4 ± 1.5	0.237
Cognition impairment	1.0 [0.0–5.0]	2.5 [0.0–5.5]	1.0 [0.0–5.0]	0.456	2.0 [0.0–5.0]	4.5 [0.5–6.0]	2.0 [0.0–5.0]	0.389
Total score	8.0 [5.0–1.5]	12.5 [6.5–15.0]	8.0 [5.5–12.0]	0.053	9.2 ± 4.4	13.1 ± 4.7	9.4 ± 4.5	0.016 *

Data are expressed as the frequency (proportion), mean with standard deviation, and median with the interquartile range (IQR). Differences that are statistically significant are indicated with an asterisk, signifying a *p*-value of less than 0.05. HGS, handgrip strength.

4. Discussion

In this study, we investigated the predictive ability of the JHFRAT in older patients who were transferred to a rehabilitation ward for stroke in a tertiary university hospital. In the ROC curve analysis, the JHFRAT demonstrated good overall diagnostic accuracy in the group with a low HGS (AUC = 0.74), whereas its performance in the entire cohort was slightly lower (AUC = 0.67). The total JHFRAT score did not significantly differ according to whether a patient had experienced falls. However, when we re-analyzed the group with a low HGS, the total JHFRAT score was significantly higher among patients that experienced falls, and within individual items, both intestinal/urinary excretion issues and the use of drugs that pose a high risk of falls were significantly higher among patients that had experienced falls. This study is clinically significant as it presents, for the first time, the efficacy of the JHFRAT in predicting falls among older individuals during the subacute phase following a stroke within a rehabilitation ward setting. Furthermore, the JHFRAT, a tool commonly used in tertiary hospitals to assess the fall risk of general acute care patients, was validated for use in the older population with stroke. Particularly, from our results, when analyzing only individuals with a low HGS, the JHFRAT exhibited higher accuracy and utility in predicting falls than it did in the overall cohort.

Muscle weakness is a significant risk factor for falls [8,29]. A low HGS is generally reported as an indicator of overall muscle strength [30] and does not only increase the fall risk of older adults [11] but also serves as a predictor of dynamic postural balance [31]. In a meta-analysis of prospective cohort studies, HGS was associated with a 53% higher risk of falls [10]. Furthermore, the proportion of patients with a low HGS on the unaffected side was high (77.1%) in our study cohort. We posit that older people with a low HGS on the unaffected side are at a higher risk of falling than the general older population. Our results indicate that a low muscle strength is associated with fall risk and may spur the development of more effective and up-to-date fall prevention strategies for older individuals.

The reported fall rate is approximately 20% for older individuals admitted to the rehabilitation ward [32]. In a study conducted at the stroke rehabilitation ward of a geriatric clinic in Sweden, 36% of patients experienced falls during the initial 8 weeks of rehabilitation, with 22% falling more than once [3]. In the present study, we identified an overall fall incidence of 6.9% among older individuals, with a rate of 5.9% observed among those with a low HGS during the subacute stroke phase within the rehabilitation ward. This relatively lower fall rate may be attributed to the thorough fall prevention education provided to patients and their caregivers (the previous study was conducted nearly 30 years ago), as well as the effective fall prevention strategy implemented by experienced nursing staff in the rehabilitation ward in a tertiary hospital setting.

A previous review of factors associated with falls during post-stroke rehabilitation emphasized the scarcity and variability of evidence concerning the influence of demographic variables, current health status, medication use, functional and sensory deficits, cognitive and perceptual impairments, and physical capabilities in relation to falls [33]. In this study, we also discovered no significant differences in either general or stroke-specific risk factors based on the occurrence of falls. Although no differences in baseline characteristics according to falls were observed in either the overall cohort or the group with a low HGS, the duration of acute treatment was significantly longer among those who experienced falls than among those who did not. This observation is notable because neither stroke severity nor the presence of stroke-specific impairments differed between patients who experienced falls and those who did not among patients with a low HGS. We infer that medical conditions following stroke, rather than stroke-specific impairments, may be the primary factors that contributed to the observed difference.

This study is the first in which the JHFRAT was analyzed specifically among older patients with stroke in a rehabilitation ward. Therefore, directly comparing fall predictions using the AUC with those in other studies may be challenging. However, other studies in which the JHFRAT was analyzed in older inpatients yielded similar results. For instance,

Hur et al. reported an AUC of 0.61 for hospitalized patients aged 65 years and older in their study in Korea [24]. A validation study of the JHFRAT among older hospitalized patients in the Netherlands revealed an overall AUC of 0.67, which varied between 0.62 and 0.71 over different 6-month intervals [34]. In the group with a low HGS in this study, the overall predictive ability of the JHFRAT was higher than that in the overall cohort, and its predictive ability was acceptable in both groups. This indicates that the use of the JHFRAT is particularly valuable in the prediction of falls in older patients with stroke and a low HGS, who represent a more fragile patient group. According to the Youden index, the optimal cutoff score for the overall cohort was 11, whereas that for the group with a low HGS was 12. In the low-HGS subgroup, setting the cutoff score at 6 resulted in the highest sensitivity (100%) and a specificity of 24%. On the other hand, with an optimal cutoff score of 12, the sensitivity and specificity were 75% and 72%, respectively, and with a cutoff score of 13, they were 62% and 77%, respectively.

Among older adults with a low HGS, those who had experienced falls had significantly higher total JHFRAT scores. Among the individual components of the JHFRAT, these patients had a significantly higher prevalence of problems related to bowel and urinary elimination, as well as a significantly higher use of drugs posing a high risk of falls. A previous study conducted in a rehabilitation ward with older patients with stroke, similar to ours, yielded similar fall predictors. Consistent with our results, Nyberg and Gustafson identified the presence of urinary incontinence and the use of diuretics, antidepressants, or sedatives as potential fall risks, alongside other clinical risk factors [3]. Urinary incontinence is a common geriatric syndrome. According to a meta-analysis, it affects up to 34% of men and up to 50% of women aged 60 years and above [35]. Consistent with our results, a recent study revealed that older adults (aged $\geq$ 65 years) with urinary incontinence were 59% more likely to experience falls than those without urinary incontinence [36]. In addition, older adults are at a markedly high risk of falls due to polypharmacy and the use of fall-risk-increasing drugs [37]. Several drug types are often referred to as "fall risk-increasing drugs," a category including antihypertensive agents, diuretics, β-blockers, sedatives and hypnotics, neuroleptics and antipsychotics, antidepressants, benzodiazepines, narcotics, and nonsteroidal anti-inflammatory drugs [38]. We discovered that the use of such medications according to the JHFRAT significantly differed between patients who had experienced falls and those who had not only among those with a low HGS. This suggests that individuals with a low HGS are more susceptible to the effects of fall-risk-increasing drugs, and that the use of all such drugs should be screened in that population.

The strength of this study lies in its presentation of the adaptability of the JHFRAT, which is typically used for hospitalized patients in the acute phase, to older individuals receiving rehabilitative care in the subacute phase of stroke recovery. However, this study also had several limitations. It was conducted at a single institution with a limited sample size, which might have limited the generalizability of the results. Additionally, the retrospective nature of the study comes with inherent limitations, such as selection bias. Furthermore, as the primary objective of this research was to evaluate the predictive accuracy of the JHFRAT among geriatric patients hospitalized after stroke, we could not use multivariable models to adjust for potential confounding factors, as the incidence of falls within the study cohort was small. However, our study was focused on a homogeneous group of patients aged $\geq$65 years in the same department after experiencing a stroke. Additionally, the baseline characteristics did not differ between those who experienced falls and those who did not. To address the abovementioned limitations, future research should involve larger and more diverse populations, possibly across multiple centers, and long-term follow-up studies should be conducted to validate and expand our results.

5. Conclusions

This study demonstrated the predictive validity of the JHFRAT in assessing the fall risk of older patients undergoing rehabilitation during the subacute stroke phase. The

JHFRAT, commonly used for such assessment in general acute care patients, has proven to be applicable and beneficial in the older population recovering from stroke. Furthermore, our results indicate that the JHFRAT has good diagnostic accuracy, particularly among patients with a low HGS. Although the performance of the tool in the overall cohort was slightly poorer, it was still considered adequate. These results highlight the importance of tailoring fall risk assessment tools to specific patient subgroups for more effective fall prevention strategies in clinical settings.

Author Contributions: Conceptualization, Y.-A.C.; data curation, S.H. and Y.-A.C.; formal analysis, Y.-A.C.; funding acquisition, Y.-A.C.; investigation, S.H., J.-S.K. and Y.-A.C.; methodology, Y.-A.C.; resources, J.-S.K. and Y.-A.C.; supervision, Y.-A.C.; writing—original draft, S.H. and Y.-A.C.; writing—review and editing, Y.-A.C. All authors have read and agreed to the published version of the manuscript.

Funding: This research was supported by the Basic Science Research Program through the National Research Foundation of Korea (NRF) funded by the Ministry of Education (2021R1I1A1A01040270).

Institutional Review Board Statement: This study was approved by the institutional review board of the tertiary hospital (IRB number: OC23RISI0119, approval date: 27 October 2023), and all methods were performed in accordance with the Code of Ethics of the World Medical Association (Declaration of Helsinki).

Informed Consent Statement: Owing to the retrospective nature of the study, the need for patient consent was waived by the IRB.

Data Availability Statement: All data analyzed during this study are available from the corresponding author upon reasonable request, owing to privacy restrictions.

Conflicts of Interest: The authors have no conflicts of interest to declare. The funders had no role in the design of the study; in the collection, analyses, or interpretation of data; in the writing of the manuscript; or in the decision to publish the results.

eferences

W.H.O. Falls. Available online: https://www.who.int/news-room/fact-sheets/detail/falls (accessed on 20 December 2023).

Hauer, K.; Lamb, S.E.; Jorstad, E.C.; Todd, C.; Becker, C.; PROFANE-Group. Systematic review of definitions and methods of measuring falls in randomised controlled fall prevention trials. *Age Ageing* **2006**, *35*, 5–10. [CrossRef]

Nyberg, L.; Gustafson, Y. Patient falls in stroke rehabilitation: A challenge to rehabilitation strategies. *Stroke* **1995**, *26*, 838–842. [CrossRef] [PubMed]

Vaishya, R.; Vaish, A. Falls in older adults are serious. *Indian J. Orthop.* **2020**, *54*, 69–74. [CrossRef]

Tinetti, M.E.; Speechley, M.; Ginter, S.F. Risk factors for falls among elderly persons living in the community. *N. Engl. J. Med.* **1988**, *319*, 1701–1707. [CrossRef]

Graafmans, W.C.; Ooms, M.E.; Hofstee, H.M.; Bezemer, P.D.; Bouter, L.M.; Lips, P. Falls in the elderly: A prospective study of risk factors and risk profiles. *Am. J. Epidemiol.* **1996**, *143*, 1129–1136. [CrossRef] [PubMed]

Jalayondeja, C.; Sullivan, P.E.; Pichaiyongwongdee, S. Six-month prospective study of fall risk factors identification in patients post-stroke. *Geriatr. Gerontol. Int.* **2014**, *14*, 778–785. [CrossRef] [PubMed]

Liu, H.; Hou, Y.; Li, H.; Lin, J. Influencing factors of weak grip strength and fall: A study based on the China Health and Retirement Longitudinal Study (CHARLS). *BMC Public Health* **2022**, *22*, 2337. [CrossRef]

Neri, S.G.R.; Lima, R.M.; Ribeiro, H.S.; Vainshelboim, B. Poor handgrip strength determined clinically is associated with falls in older women. *J. Frailty Sarcopenia Falls* **2021**, *6*, 43–49. [CrossRef]

). Moreland, J.D.; Richardson, J.A.; Goldsmith, C.H.; Clase, C.M. Muscle weakness and falls in older adults: A systematic review and meta-analysis. *J. Am. Geriatr. Soc.* **2004**, *52*, 1121–1129. [CrossRef]

.. Bobowik, P.; Wiszomirska, I. Diagnostic dependence of muscle strength measurements and the risk of falls in the elderly. *Int. J. Rehabil. Res.* **2020**, *43*, 330–336. [CrossRef]

2. Maulden, S.A.; Gassaway, J.; Horn, S.D.; Smout, R.J.; DeJong, G. Timing of initiation of rehabilitation after stroke. *Arch. Phys. Med. Rehabil.* **2005**, *86* (Suppl. 2), S34–S40. [CrossRef] [PubMed]

3. Cumbler, E.U.; Simpson, J.R.; Rosenthal, L.D.; Likosky, D.J. Inpatient falls: Defining the problem and identifying possible solutions. Part I: An evidence-based review. *Neurohospitalist* **2013**, *3*, 135–143. [CrossRef] [PubMed]

4. Joint Commission International, International Patient Safety Goals [Online]. Joint Commission International. 2017. Available online: https://www.jointcommissioninternational.org/improve/international-patient-safety-goals/ (accessed on 21 December 2023).

15. Chen, Y.; Lv, L.; Wu, C.; Wen, H.; Cai, H.; Xiao, Y.; Zhu, H. Assessment of the predictive ability of the Johns Hopkins Fall Ris Assessment Tool (Chinese Version) in inpatient settings. *J. Adv. Nurs.* **2022**, *78*, 4054–4061. [CrossRef] [PubMed]
16. Poe, S.S.; Dawson, P.B.; Cvach, M.; Burnett, M.; Kumble, S.; Lewis, M.; Thompson, C.B.; Hill, E.E. The johns Hopkins fall ris assessment tool: A Study of Reliability and Validity. *J. Nurs. Care Qual.* **2018**, *33*, 10–19. [CrossRef] [PubMed]
17. Kim, K.S.; Kim, J.A.; Choi, Y.K.; Kim, Y.J.; Park, M.H.; Kim, H.Y.; Song, M.S. A comparative study on the validity of fall ris assessment scales in Korean hospitals. *Asian Nurs. Res. (Korean Soc. Nurs. Sci.)* **2011**, *5*, 28–37. [CrossRef]
18. Cox, R.; Buckholtz, B.; Bradas, C.; Bowden, V.; Kerber, K.; McNett, M.M. Risk factors for falls among hospitalized acu post–ischemic stroke patients. *J. Neurosci. Nurs.* **2017**, *49*, 355–360. [CrossRef] [PubMed]
19. Suzuki, T.; Sonoda, S.; Misawa, K.; Saitoh, E.; Shimizu, Y.; Kotake, T. Incidence and consequence of falls in inpatient rehabilitatio of stroke patients. *Exp. Aging Res.* **2005**, *31*, 457–469. [CrossRef] [PubMed]
20. Teasell, R.; McRae, M.; Foley, N.; Bhardwaj, A. The incidence and consequences of falls in stroke patients during inpatier rehabilitation: Factors associated with high risk. *Arch. Phys. Med. Rehabil.* **2002**, *83*, 329–333. [CrossRef] [PubMed]
21. Persson, C.U.; Kjellberg, S.; Lernfelt, B.; Westerlind, E.; Cruce, M.; Hansson, P.O. Risk of falling in a stroke unit after acute strok The Fall Study of Gothenburg (FallsGOT). *Clin. Rehabil.* **2018**, *32*, 398–409. [CrossRef]
22. Czernuszenko, A.; Członkowska, A. Risk factors for falls in stroke patients during inpatient rehabilitation. *Clin. Rehabil.* **2009**, 2 176–188. [CrossRef]
23. Dudzińska-Griszek, J.; Szuster, K.; Szewieczek, J. Grip strength as a frailty diagnostic component in geriatric inpatients. *Cli Interv. Aging* **2017**, *12*, 1151–1157. [CrossRef]
24. Hur, E.Y.; Jin, Y.; Jin, T.; Lee, S.M. Longitudinal evaluation of Johns Hopkins fall risk assessment tool and nurses' experience. *Nurs. Care Qual.* **2017**, *32*, 242–251. [CrossRef]
25. Chen, L.K.; Woo, J.; Assantachai, P.; Auyeung, T.W.; Chou, M.Y.; Iijima, K.; Jang, H.C.; Kang, L.; Kim, M.; Kim, S.; et al. Asia Working Group for Sarcopenia: 2019 consensus update on sarcopenia diagnosis and treatment. *J. Am. Med. Dir. Assoc.* **2020**, 2 300–307.e2. [CrossRef] [PubMed]
26. Nyberg, L.; Gustafson, Y. Fall prediction index for patients in stroke rehabilitation. *Stroke* **1997**, *28*, 716–721. [CrossRef] [PubMec
27. Yeung, S.S.Y.; Reijnierse, E.M.; Pham, V.K.; Trappenburg, M.C.; Lim, W.K.; Meskers, C.G.M.; Maier, A.B. Sarcopenia and it association with falls and fractures in older adults: A systematic review and meta-analysis. *J. Cachexia Sarcopenia Muscle* **2019**, 1 485–500. [CrossRef] [PubMed]
28. Hajian-Tilaki, K. Receiver operating characteristic (ROC) curve analysis for medical diagnostic test evaluation. *Caspian J. Inter Med.* **2013**, *4*, 627–635.
29. Centers for Disease Control and Prevention. Preventing Falls: A Guide to Implementing Effective Community-Based Fa Prevention Programs. Available online: https://www.cdc.gov/falls/programs/community_prevention.html (accessed on 2 December 2023).
30. Beaudart, C.; Rolland, Y.; Cruz-Jentoft, A.J.; Bauer, J.M.; Sieber, C.; Cooper, C.; Al-Daghri, N.; Araujo de Carvalho, I.; Bautmans, I Bernabei, R.; et al. Assessment of muscle function and physical performance in daily clinical practice: A position paper endorse by the European Society for Clinical and Economic Aspects of Osteoporosis, Osteoarthritis and Musculoskeletal Diseases (ESCEO *Calcif. Tissue. Int.* **2019**, *105*, 1–14. [CrossRef]
31. Alonso, A.C.; Ribeiro, S.M.; Luna, N.M.S.; Peterson, M.D.; Bocalini, D.S.; Serra, M.M.; Brech, G.C.; Greve, J.M.D.A.; Garcez-Leme L.E. Association between handgrip strength, balance, and knee flexion/extension strength in older adults. *PLoS ONE* **2018**, *1* e0198185. [CrossRef]
32. Vassallo, M.; Sharma, J.C.; Briggs, R.S.; Allen, S.C. Characteristics of early fallers on elderly patient rehabilitation wards. *Ag Ageing* **2003**, *32*, 338–342. [CrossRef]
33. Campbell, G.B.; Matthews, J.T. An integrative review of factors associated with falls during post-stroke rehabilitation. *J. Nur Scholarsh.* **2010**, *42*, 395–404. [CrossRef]
34. Damoiseaux-Volman, B.A.; van Schoor, N.M.; Medlock, S.; Romijn, J.A.; van der Velde, N.; Abu-Hanna, A. External validation o the Johns Hopkins Fall Risk Assessment Tool in older Dutch hospitalized patients. *Eur. Geriatr. Med.* **2023**, *14*, 69–77. [CrossRef [PubMed]
35. John, G.; Bardini, C.; Combescure, C.; Dällenbach, P. Urinary incontinence as a predictor of death: A systematic review anc meta-analysis. *PLoS ONE* **2016**, *11*, e0158992. [CrossRef] [PubMed]
36. Moon, S.; Chung, H.S.; Kim, Y.J.; Kim, S.J.; Kwon, O.; Lee, Y.G.; Yu, J.M.; Cho, S.T. The impact of urinary incontinence on falls: A systematic review and meta-analysis. *PLoS ONE* **2021**, *16*, e0251711. [CrossRef] [PubMed]
37. World Health Organization. Medication Safety in Polypharmacy [Technical Report]. Available online: https://iris.who.int handle/10665/325454 (accessed on 21 December 2023).
38. Woolcott, J.C.; Richardson, K.J.; Wiens, M.O.; Patel, B.; Marin, J.; Khan, K.M.; Marra, C.A. Meta-analysis of the impact of 9 medication classes on falls in elderly persons. *Arch. Intern. Med.* **2009**, *169*, 1952–1960. [CrossRef] [PubMed]

MDPI AG
Grosspeteranlage 5
4052 Basel
Switzerland
Tel.: +41 61 683 77 34

Healthcare Editorial Office
E-mail: healthcare@mdpi.com
www.mdpi.com/journal/healthcare

www.ingramcontent.com/pod-product-compliance
Lightning Source LLC
LaVergne TN
LVHW070444061126
851858LV00011B/161
* 9 7 8 3 7 2 5 8 7 9 2 3 6 *